CANCER

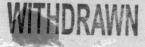

Cancer

What every patient needs to know

DR. JEFFREY TOBIAS

BLOOMSBURY

To my parents,
With love and gratitude

First published in 1995 by Bloomsbury Publishing plc, 2 Soho Square,
London W1V 6HB

Copyright © by Dr. Jeffrey Tobias

The moral right of the author has been asserted

British Library Cataloguing in Publication Data

A CIP record for this book is available from the British Library

ISBN 0 7475 1993 5

10 9 8 7 6 5 4 3 2 1

Typeset by Hewer Text Composition Services, Edinburgh
Printed and bound in Great Britain by Cox & Wyman Ltd, Reading, Berkshire

CONTENTS

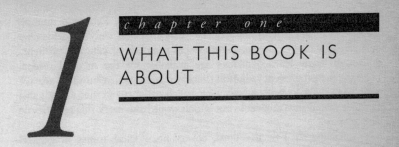

chapter one

WHAT THIS BOOK IS ABOUT

Introduction

I spend most of my professional time looking after patients with cancer, with research, teaching and administration filling the free moments. After almost twenty years as a cancer specialist, first as trainee and now as a consultant, I have written or edited several books and a hundred or so specialist articles for the profession; I now think that it is high time the general public had their own book on cancer, written by a specialist.

It seems to me a good time to attempt this. In the first place, we now talk about cancer ever more openly, with far less inhibition and dogma than before and, by and large, with as much candour as in other branches of medicine. Secondly, cancer medicine moves at a remarkably rapid rate, and new treatments are increasingly pounced upon by the media, almost before the ink is dry on the first research paper. For both patients and doctors, this can have alarming consequences. Thirdly, there is increasing public concern at the restricted availability of top-class facilities for cancer in the UK, and of the relatively small number of specialists we have. The Royal Colleges and other senior medical groups have made no secret of this, and are themselves acting as pressure groups to try and improve matters. All this means that patients with cancer are likely to have only a restricted period of time with the specialist they are referred to, so many will need advice as to how best to use this time and what important

1

questions they might wish to ask. Finally, 1995 is the centenary year of the discovery of radium by Marie and Pierre Curie. Radiation therapy was used for cancer within a very few years after that truly historic event and remains one of the most important methods of cancer treatment. Although many learned articles are available for the medical reader, charting the progress of radiation therapy during its first hundred years, I wanted to make a small contribution which patients and their friends and families would find accessible but which would also mark this remarkable anniversary.

Approximately half the book covers oncological topics of general interest: causes, genetic predisposition, the sometimes baffling differences in cancer prevalence in various parts of the world, and so on. The remainder of the book covers the specific cancers in more detail, with an emphasis on the commonest types, their different patterns of behaviour and an account of the main approaches to treatment for each. Current areas of cancer research cannot be covered in detail, but the extremely important concept of clinical trials for cancer is discussed at length, since it has such bearing on all our lives. It is also, as it happens, one of the most important ways by which a cancer patient can contribute to the future well-being of other sufferers with the same complaint, as well as assuring him or herself of the highest standards of treatment. Finally, there is a brief description of the work of the hospice movement, together with an account of the important principles of continuing and terminal care for patients with cancer who cannot be cured and are likely to be close to the end of their lives. Even as little as ten years ago, this whole area was still taboo; many patients are now happy to talk more openly about this most distressing aspect of their illness. Many more are dying at home, ably supported not only by their general practitioners, but also by dedicated teams of Macmillan nurses or, in some cases, multi-disciplinary groups of nurses, doctors, counsellors, and social workers. Patients suffering from chronic disorders other than cancer often remark wryly that cancer patients are so much better off than they! I can see there is some truth in it.

Many patients who have cancer do indeed write about it; in fact, many of the books available are courageous and sometimes shocking accounts of a personal journey which, though sometimes ending in tragedy, is often also uplifting. I have very great respect for many of these, but they could hardly be expected to provide a dispassionate account of the subject, or deal with many of the details which other patients will want to know about. There are other books by paramedics or counsellors, some of which I find myself somewhat dubious about. It can be galling for a specialist who has spent years, perhaps decades, studying for specialist exams, seeing and supporting desperately ill patients and trying to think creatively about possible new approaches, to read accounts by individuals who have had little or no specialist training, have no professional body to answer to, and sometimes seem to be taking their vulnerable subjects or clients for a ride. I don't, of course, wish to tar all such advisors or groups with the same brush, and I am not so arrogant to believe there is nothing that medical specialists can learn from them. What worries me, however, is the relatively uncritical way in which many of them press their pet remedy and the ease with which a vulnerable, sometimes desperate, patient (or parent, partner or friend) can be carried along on a wave of sometimes misplaced enthusiasm. Chapters 9 and 11 deal with this issue much more fully, but this seems a good place to put on record my general feelings about this difficult issue.

Few things give more professional pleasure than talking to a patient in the consulting room – preferably a lively debate with plenty of cut and thrust if the patient has ideas of his (or her) own, and doesn't wish simply to be a passive recipient of the doctor's advice. I don't mind being questioned, disagreed with or asked if I'd mind another opinion being sought. What I do find hard to swallow, however, is the extraordinary loss of critical faculties which some patients display when attending an 'alternative' practitioner, who might offer diet, reflexology, iridotherapy, aromatherapy, colour therapy and a host of other approaches with little, if any, scientific enquiry or justification to support their use. Fortunately, the most extreme examples of these techniques seem less prevalent than a few years ago, and both conventional doctors like myself and the 'alternative' practitioners have settled down to a less argumentative position, to the benefit, I think, of most of our patients. In the bad old days, I was certainly aware of unscrupulous alternative groups, who argued strongly that patients should avoid conventional treatment altogether; this is much less common now. Conventional doctors, for their part, mostly now take the view that if the patient wishes to augment the cancer treatment by dietary or other means, this may at the very least be a useful way by which they can make a contribution to their own recovery rather than remaining at the receiving end of treatment. However, I still get worried by some of the more excluding food fads (see chapter 11).

What this book sets out to do is to try and demystify first of all the subject itself (both the general issues relating to cancer and also some of the specifics) and, in addition to empower patients as far as humanly possible. The word 'cancer' still carries many of the traditional connotations, despite the increased openness I referred to earlier – the shock, the helplessness, the enervating anxiety. Yet more and more patients are being cured, treatment side-effects are being reduced, cancer pain and other symptoms are generally controllable. Many patients live highly active lives, in many cases even after relapse and further treatment have reduced the chance of a complete cure. I return to this in chapter 7.

To all of you, I want to say this: don't let the cancer become the central focus of your life. You still have an important contribution to make, whether at work, as a member of your family (perhaps a parent, husband, wife, whatever). You're not alone, though you might feel it at times. Many of you will decide not to say anything at all at work, others will be more public about it. You don't need to feel that you 'ought' to deal with it in any other way than whatever comes naturally. If your inclination is to be cautious before telling too many others at work, don't be swayed by well-meaning friends who insist that 'you have to talk about it' to all and sundry. It certainly doesn't help keeping such weighty news to yourself entirely, but there is no set formula, no clear yardstick, to tell you how to react. I've known patients choose an entirely private path, firmly and calmly believing that they will come through best that way (sometimes they are right); others shout, scream or hit the bottle in a genuine need to rail against the unfairness of it all. It can be wearing for all concerned, but if that's what you need, do it! Don't worry too much about the poor embattled friend or partner trying to cope with it all – this is one time in your life when you really do have to put yourself first. You may even gain from the experience – I know plenty of patients who have.

Not even the most optimistic of specialists (and I admit I probably fall into that category) would pretend that having cancer is generally a positive or pleasurable experience, but for the fortunate ones who are cured, or have many comfortable years before the return of the disease, there can be undoubted benefits. Many see themselves in a rather new light and recognise new priorities which put previous concerns in a more realistic perspective. Many recognise, and some for the first time, that there are more important things than the colour of the bedroom walls or the size and engine capacity of the new car. Doing what you've always put off, spending more time with family or friends that have been taken for granted for too long, fulfilling private ambitions – these are a few of the changes many people make in their lives. Others, perhaps the most fortunate of all, realise that they're happy continuing in the same old way, but perhaps with a greater sense of satisfaction than before. Maybe it's lack of imagination, but most patients, even those faced with a relatively short prognosis (probable survival time), make few obvious changes in their lives, but live the final months with greater personal intensity.

I well remember one patient who startled me by saying, a few years after he had been diagnosed, that his cancer was the best thing that ever happened to him – not something that patients say to you every day. This was a twenty-three-year-old single man who, following investigations for infertility, was found to be suffering from a testicular tumour. It was removed surgically, leaving the other intact, and as the scans and tumour markers were all clear (see chapter 17) no further treatment was required. However, whilst in hospital having the orchidectomy (surgical removal of the testicle), he met a rather attractive staff nurse who turned out to be the girl of his dreams. They later married, and ten years on, I have discharged him from the clinic, completely cured. True, he lost a testicle, but as he has pointed out to me several times, he's always got the other one and it's never yet let him down.

On a personal level, you must do what you think is right, but for heaven's sake get yourself as well informed as possible. I hope this book helps you to achieve that, in conjunction with the advice you'll doubtless receive from the specialist looking after you. It is not by any means my intention to undermine what he or she will advise, but there may, of course, be areas where we appear to disagree. So ask! There is likely to be a good reason for any apparent inconsistency of view. Despite the extreme pressure British specialists are working under, oncologists (cancer doctors), surgeons and others treating cancer in the UK are trained to an extremely high standard and are amongst the very finest in the world. I was on a television panel recently in which the question asked was, 'Can you trust your doctor?' In my view, the answer is an emphatic 'Yes', though inevitably one can always find anecdotes where the standard of care has fallen short. If you really feel that you can't go along with what the specialist is advising, you can always seek a second opinion. Don't forget that all the changes in our newly commercialised health service are supposed to flow from the concept of 'patient power'. Don't be too easily cowed. Who knows, your specialist might even prefer it that way as well. I know I certainly do.

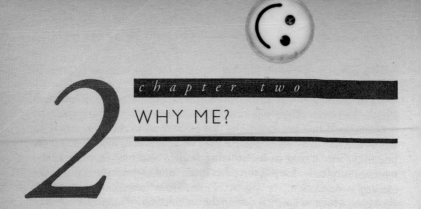

chapter two

WHY ME?

What we know about the causes of cancer

All too often, we have little or no idea what might have caused a cancer to develop in the first place or, to be more accurate, what might have triggered the initial malignant change. Just as with known potential causes of heart disease – high blood pressure, lack of exercise, the wrong kind of food and so on – cancer is clearly a multifactorial illness in terms of its causes or origins. It's almost never true that a single cancer-triggering insult is the sole initiator of such complex biological processes. Even more baffling, perhaps, is the curious chain of events that might lead a cancer to redevelop as secondary tumours distant from the primary site, at a much later stage, after apparent cure of the initial tumour by surgical removal or radiotherapy. The biology of these events is only poorly understood.

We do, however, have many clues, mostly in the form of cancer genetics, epidemiology, and cancer carcinogenesis (the chain of events leading towards malignant change), all specific areas within the study of causation of cancer. Our ever-increasing understanding of these various influences seems to me a fine example of the type of bridge-building between previously disparate specialities which often marks the most valuable types of original research.

CANCER GENETICS

There is no doubt that some families have a genetic predisposition to cancer, with some family members developing cancers of a particular type (breast cancer is a good example) and others experiencing a variety of malignant changes which might truly type such a cluster as a 'cancer family'. In families such as these, there seems little doubt that genetic predisposition is a real event, even though many of the cancers may be common, so coincidental clustering could occur simply as a matter of chance. A number of features might, however, suggest that in any individual patient a developing cancer really does have a strong genetic background. These are generally thought to include unusual tumours occurring in two or more close relatives, or a commoner type of cancer occurring at a younger age than normal.

In addition, there are a number of well known syndromes, often very complicated ones, in which an inherited abnormality through a chromosomal irregularity, such as Down's syndrome, predisposes such individuals to a higher risk of certain cancers than one would normally expect. In recent years, many of these have become far better characterised, with both the precise chromosomal abnormality, and the degree of cancer risk, now known in better detail. In Down's syndrome, for example, there is an extra chromosomal fragment at position 21, leading not only to a particular appearance of the individuals, but also to an increased incidence of acute leukaemia, which not infrequently is the cause of death at a relatively young age. Another good example is that of 'familial adenomatous polyposis' (FAP), an inherited disorder in which individuals suffer from multiple colonic (large bowel) polyps and other specific abnormalities, eventually developing colonic or other carcinomas which may prove fatal. The cause of this is now recognised as a specific abnormality on the 5q chromosome, and affected individuals are often advised to undergo total resection of the large bowel in order to prevent the potentially fatal cancer developing. Unappealing, perhaps, but frequently a life-saving operation.

Overall, up to ten per cent of common cancers, particularly those of breast, ovary and large bowel, appear to occur in familial clusters, with a predisposition in these families to a single, dominant, inherited gene, and with the implication that any children of an affected patient have a fifty per cent risk or more of inheriting this increased risk of cancer. However, because of the multifactorial nature of cancer development mentioned above, it does not then follow that all these patients will in due course develop a malignant tumour. This depends on many other factors, such as the power or penetrance of the genetic predisposition, and probably on dietary and other lifestyle factors as well.

Very few cancers occur solely as a result of genetic predisposition, but in the rare childhood cancer, retinoblastoma, which is a malignant disease of the eye occurring in very young children, there is a powerful familial component, and the genetics are reasonably well understood. The rate of this tumour appears to have doubled over the past fifty years, largely due to affected children surviving and having children themselves, many of whom will then be affected. It is inherited by an autosomal (i.e. non-sex linked) dominant gene, and the offspring of survivors of hereditary retinoblastoma (i.e. those with a positive family history) will themselves have a fifty per cent chance of developing the tumour. This also seems to apply to the much less common, sporadic (i.e. non-familial) but bilateral (both eyes affected) case. Survivors of unilateral (one-sided), sporadic cases have a ten per cent chance or so of themselves having an affected child, so these parents, though not themselves from retinoblastoma families, must presumably have been 'silent carriers'.

With modern treatment methods, most of the affected children can be cured without serious loss of vision, since radiotherapy and chemotherapy are often at least as effective as surgery. This success story serves well to illustrate the importance of genetic identification and predisposition, and the number of known cases of genetically linked, common cancers does seem to be growing.

EPIDEMIOLOGY OF CANCER

Epidemiology is the study of populations, their habits, types of illness, dietary preferences and so on. Studies of cancer epidemiology, comparing different rates of cancer development in different parts of the world or perhaps in different socio-economic groups, have been extremely productive in our understanding of the process of cancer development. Obviously the possibility arises that certain foods, behaviour patterns or other aspects of lifestyle might be responsible for the extraordinary differences that occur, though genetics may also play a part. The situation is further complicated by the frequency of migration and settlement we see so often nowadays. By and large, however, migrating populations tend to develop the cancer-risk pattern of their new home, suggesting, perhaps, that genetics may be less important than environmental influences.

Epidemiological studies have been extremely powerful in determining changes of cancer incidence in different countries throughout the sixty-year period from the 1930s, an era in which accurate record keeping has become established in most Western European countries and North America. From these studies, we know, for example, that breast and testicular cancer continue to rise in incidence and that cancer of the stomach is clearly on the decline. For breast cancer, we know that, aside from familial predisposition, important factors include age at first pregnancy (the younger the woman is, the less likely she is to develop the cancer), with a three times greater likelihood of breast cancer development for women bearing their first child over the age of thirty compared with those who are under the age of twenty at first pregnancy.

With changing social attitudes, better contraception and increased numbers of women seeking careers, which may delay their first pregnancy until this age, this one feature alone could account for the ten per cent increase in the incidence of breast cancer that was noted in both the UK and USA in the 1970s and early 1980s. Even now, the incidence of breast cancer appears to be rising in many Western countries, by about two per cent per annum. Breast cancer has become so common in the Western world that one in ten women are now expected to develop it at some point during their lifetime, with even greater prevalence figures in certain parts of the country. In some parts of the USA, the figure is one in eight. In testicular cancer, the rise in incidence over the past twenty-five years remains largely unexplained, though some authorities believe that the fall in the average male sperm count, possibly related to environmental factors, could in some way be related.

Lung cancer is a particularly fascinating and tragic example of a tumour in which we know almost all we need to know about causation, in order to eradicate it altogether (or very nearly); yet this common and often fatal tumour remains the main cause of cancer death in most parts of Europe and the USA. The strength of the data linking cigarette smoking to lung cancer can hardly be over-emphasised. In both males and females, the rise in incidence of lung cancer was preceded (by about twenty years) by a sharp rise in cigarette smoking, first in men between 1910 and 1940, and latterly in women between about 1940 and 1960. In the 1950s, the male:female ratio for lung cancer was about ten to one, whereas the figure now is less than three to one, simply as a result of the women catching up. Clearly, advertising campaigns targeted at women have been hugely successful, with the appalling result that lung cancer in women, once uncommon, is now among the more frequent malignant tumours, even in relatively young women in their forties and fifties. In a well-studied population of British professional classes (mostly doctors), the falling proportion of smokers has been accompanied by a real reduction in the probability of their developing lung cancer. We also have two more powerful pieces of information that genuinely quantify the risk between cigarette smoke and the development of lung cancer; firstly the clear relationship between the number of cigarettes smoked per day and the relative risk of developing lung cancer, and secondly, the clear indication that, after twelve to fifteen years of abstinence from cigarette smoking, the risk of developing the cancer falls to such a low level that it is almost as if the ex-smoker had never smoked at all!

Why do different populations have such widely differing rates of cancer incidence? Some groups smoke more, some less. In the USA, the incidence of lung cancer among professional white males has fallen recently (the first time ever that the fall was documented in a large population group other than the specific example of British doctors), whereas in other parts of the world, particularly China and the Far East, lung cancer rates continue to rise as smoking becomes more prevalent with little or no attempt at educating the population.

For other types of cancer, lifestyle and dietary differences appear to be closely linked with the development of a particular cancer, though the causal relationship is far less clear than that between, say, cigarette smoking and lung cancer. Studies have been carried out which chart the relationship between fat intake and the development of breast cancer, and between intake of dietary meat protein and the development of cancer of the large bowel. There is a clear relationship in each of these cases, yet is the definable characteristic – the meat in one case, the fat in the other – truly the causative agent? Could it not be that, in each of these cases, something else about an affluent lifestyle is perhaps the offending initiator of malignant change, with the fat or meat intake simply serving as a marker of, if you like, a too-affluent lifestyle which departs from some predetermined but more natural dietary state?

Carcinogenesis

Some agents, such as cigarette smoke, are clearly carcinogenic (liable to cause a cancerous change), but what is it within them that is the real culprit? Is it possible to produce a really safe cigarette by excluding the dangerous chemical? And what about the biological processes that take place within the cell when a cancer change is triggered?

In the case of lung cancer, many of the constituents of cigarette smoke are thought to be carcinogenic, including nicotine itself, trace elements, and toxic, organic chemicals, such as benzpyrene and benzofluoranthenes (they even *sound* dangerous!). Other causal factors have also been implicated in lung cancer, including exposure to radioactivity from deep mining (particularly a problem in China) and an increased risk in certain industries, such as nickel refining, and in the industrial manufacture of chromium and chromate products. A particularly nasty form of lung cancer affecting the outer covering, or pleura, of the lung is clearly associated with previous exposure to asbestos. This is dealt with more fully in chapter 12.

It is also important to note that cigarette smoking doesn't only cause lung cancer. It is clearly linked to cancers of the mouth, larynx (voice box), pancreas, kidney and bladder – these latter two, presumably, because of cigarette smoke carcinogens which enter the blood stream and are concentrated in the kidney and held in the bladder for several hours at a time before finally leaving the body when the individual urinates. Cancer of the cervix is another tumour in which cigarette smoking appears to be causative. In parts of the world outside Western Europe, tobacco used in other ways can also cause cancer to develop. In India, for example, one of the commonest types of cancer occurs within the oral cavity, often at a number of sites, due to the widespread habit of retaining a tobacco-betel nut *pan* in the mouth, often throughout the day. Some Third World populations like to smoke with the lit end within the mouth, a potent cause of cancer of the palate. Oral cancer in India is the counterpart of lung cancer in the West.

Occupational exposure to dangerous chemicals should largely be a thing of the past, but in former days, it was an important clue to cancer causation. In 1775, the great Bart's surgeon, Sir Percivall Pott, noted a very high incidence of skin cancer over the scrotum in chimney sweeps, and it later turned out that some of the more unpleasant constituents of coal tar and soot had a direct effect on these poor lads, who, needless to

11

say, ended up covered from head to foot with the carcinogenic materials, though with a particularly high collection of soot and grease in their pelvic skin. About a hundred years later, it was noted that workers in dye factories had an unusually high incidence of bladder cancer, and other occupational groups were also later identified, including cable and rubber workers. We now know what some of the causative agents are 3:4 benzpyrene in coal tar (affecting the young chimney sweeps) and β-naphthylamine in the rubber and cable workers.

VIRAL CAUSES

In animals, certain viruses are known to cause cancers, and seem an increasingly likely cause of some of our human cancers as well. In China, for example, where cancer of the post-nasal space (nasopharynx) is common, there appears to be a very high level of contamination in such patients by the Epstein-Barr virus, and closer to home, many cases of cancer of the cervix are thought to be linked to a virus (as yet unidentified), possibly passed on during sexual intercourse. Certainly there is no doubt that lifelong celibate women, such as nuns, have a zero incidence of carcinoma of the cervix, whereas those with multiple partners, particularly between the ages of twelve and twenty years, are at relatively high risk. Occasional cases of husbands and wives (or partners) with, on the one hand, a carcinoma of the penis, and on the other, a cancer of the cervix, have been well documented.

For the most part, however, there is no clear-cut relationship between a viral causation and the development of human cancer, though viruses may be able to transform cells in a dangerous way, leading to a long, latent period before tumour development. This would make any link between the initiating virus and the subsequent tumour very much more difficult to confirm. Moreover, the initiating event could be an important first step, but insufficient in itself to cause a true malignant change with overt development of the cancer. Apart from the nasopharyngeal and cervical carcinomas mentioned above, other important areas where viral carcinogenesis is thought likely include Kaposi's sarcoma, the classical skin malignancy seen in so many AIDS patients, and also Burkitt's lymphoma, typically a tumour encountered in African children and adolescents, many of whom are known to be infected with the Epstein-Barr virus (though only a few of these develop the lymphoma, again a good illustration of the viral infection perhaps being necessary but not sufficient for development of the cancerous change).

RADIATION

Radiation, so valuable in the treatment of cancer (see chapter 5), is itself carcinogenic. This may seem paradoxical, but it seems clear that, at relatively low doses, radiation can damage a cell in such a way as to cause a dangerous mutation, and eventually the development of a tumour within the radiation-exposed area, whereas radiotherapy is given at much higher doses, often sufficient to kill the tumour cells entirely. Although the risk of causing a new, radiation-induced cancer is certainly one which radiotherapists are well aware of, it is generally insignificant when compared with the advantages of radiotherapy in controlling a malignant tumour which cannot easily be dealt with by other means. This risk of causing cancer is, however, an extremely good reason to withhold radiotherapy for non-malignant conditions, such as scar overgrowth in surgical wounds or chronic rheumatic disorders. Although these illnesses are rarely treated nowadays by radiotherapy (and with good reason), it is one of the more frustrating facts of medicine that some of them are extremely responsive to radiation, and many patients have had lifelong relief. One good example is the disabling, chronic stiffening of the spine known as 'ankylosing spondylitis', which generally responds to drug therapy, but which in previous times was often miraculously cured by radiation. The trouble is that, in some cases, malignant skin tumours appeared at the site of the radiation, an illustration of the very real dangers of radiation therapy when used inappropriately. Nonetheless, in some benign conditions, the risk of serious damage or death is so great that radiotherapy may be justifiable (see chapter 5).

Radiotherapy is thought to cause damage by producing breaks in strands of DNA (the double-helix genetic material discovered by Watson and Crick and present within the cell nucleus), which results in chromosomal abnormalities, such as breakage (fragmentations), complete disappearance of part of the chromosomal material (a 'deletion') and the removal of genetic material from one part of the chromosome to another (a 'translocation'). Although these changes are normally lethal to a cell, rendering it incapable of causing further trouble, they may occur to a degree which is insufficient to kill the cell, but which allows it to mutate at a later stage without the cell control mechanisms which would normally prevent a cancer from forming. It is this uncontrolled cellular growth which is generally regarded as being so dangerous.

Several types of human cancer have been documented as being more common after radiation exposure in large populations, such as occurred at Hiroshima or Chernobyl. These include thyroid cancer, leukaemia and lymphoma, and breast cancer. One fascinating fact for the cancer biologist is that it took forty years for the excess in breast cancer cases to become apparent after the Hiroshima and Nagasaki bombs in 1945, whereas the other tumour types were picked up much more rapidly. This clearly tells us something about the normal developmental biology of these different tumours. Patients so often ask, 'How long have I had it?' and, in truth, there is no easy answer, since we believe cancer is likely to have developed from a single mutant cell – and when on earth might that have taken place?

The only real clue we have to this is that a single, definable exposure to radiation in 1945 produced an increase in risk which was detectable for the first time in the mid-1980s. Does this mean that the tumour was in some way slowly developing during this whole period? Probably yes, although the other circumstances of cancer causation would affect different patients in different ways – the strength of the family history, for example. Interestingly enough, from my own case records I have a patient in her early forties without any family history of breast cancer, who developed the disease in the same year as her one other sister, a most unlikely coincidence. I probed the history further because the story was so unusual, particularly in such young patients and in such a short space of time. Interestingly, it turned out that their father had had tuberculosis when they were in their early teens, and, as contacts, they had both been subjected to an annual chest X-ray for five or six years, a practice which would not now be recommended. This would have been just at the same time as their breasts were developing, and I can't help feeling that the radiation insult of those repeated chest X-rays might have had something to do with the development (in both of them) of a breast cancer within a virtually identical time frame.

THE 'CANCER PERSONALITY'

One myth I do wish to dispel is that there is no such thing, in my view, as the 'cancer personality'. This seems to me a very dangerous concept, implying, apart from any other considerations, that at the end of the day, it was your own fault you got it in the first place! I have certainly known patients who have turned elsewhere for advice, only to be told that 'this sequence of events in your recent life, with stress, loss, inability to come to terms with the grief, etc., etc. is the cause!' I have no truck with this kind of thing. Cancer patients may be introverted, outgoing, positive or depressed. They are endlessly varied, as with all other patients, and it is, in my view, both shallow and mischievous to label them in any particular way. There is no evidence whatsoever that a particular personality type is more liable to develop cancer. It *wasn't* your fault that you got it in the first place.

There is, however, the question of why some patients are cured of cancer whereas others, with an apparently identical condition, relapse and may ultimately die from it. One celebrated study divided breast-cancer patients into four groups: the denial group (who reacted by pretending that it was happening to somebody else, not them); those who displayed 'fighting spirit' ('I'll beat it – it won't get the better of me'); the stoic acceptors, and finally the 'helpless, hopeless' group. The first two groups did far better than the latter two, and all sorts of psychological explanations were put forward to explain this phenomenon; a number of study groups are presently working on the issue. Just think, though, how difficult it is to change one's personality! If you are a natural stoic acceptor, how can you become, for example, a classic 'fighting spirit' type? It's one of those areas where I'm not sure whether knowing the results of personality studies will actually do anyone any good.

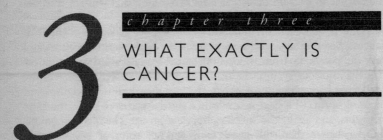

chapter three

WHAT EXACTLY IS CANCER?

ancer biology is the study of cancer evolution and development at the cellular level. As my colleague Professor Souhami has pointed out:

> *'When thinking about cancer, many scientists and physicians, and members of the public, perceive cancer as being "foreign" to the body. Analogies with infections caused by parasites and germs are often drawn, and many infectious agents have been proposed as possible triggers. As knowledge has progressed, however, it has become apparent that, in many respects, cancer cells are similar to normal cells and that there is considerable diversity of function and structure within a single neoplasm (abnormal growth). Even greater diversity exists between tumours of the same type in different individuals and between tumours of different types. The fundamental property of cancer, which distinguishes the disease from normal tissues and which makes treatment so difficult, is metastasis. We are still ignorant of the mechanisms which underlie this remarkable process.'*

Cancer is essentially the disordered and uncontrolled growth of cells within a specific organ or tissue type. Most cancers, though not all, begin in a single site, such as breast, lung or brain, and, if left untreated, grow steadily, often by invading surrounding areas (i.e. growing by direct extension), as well as producing secondary growths – the metastasis referred to by Souhami. He is right to label this as the central and most feared feature of malignant disorders, and his remark about the difficulty of treatment is the result of our inability to be certain that secondary growths are absent, and therefore unable to pose any threat to the patient's continued health and life – even after apparently successful treatment of the primary site. This uncertainty is one of the major reasons why cancer physicians are so obsessed with clinical trials (see chapter 6), since so many of our efforts are at present directed towards protecting patients, by means of whole-body (systemic) treatments, such as chemotherapy or hormones, from the possible development of these life-threatening secondary deposits of tumour.

Although most cancers originate at a single site, this is not always the case. In leukaemia, for example, the malignant transformation of blood or, more accurately, certain elements of the bone marrow which are the site of manufacture of many of the specific blood cells, the whole of the bone marrow is apparently transformed by the single initiating process which triggered the malignant change. Little is known of the causes of human leukaemia, though in animals, for example the domestic cat, a virus is known to be the cause. In other types of bone marrow cancer, notably multiple myeloma, in which a different bone marrow cell is affected, the transformed malignant areas of marrow are more patchy. Unlike leukaemia, not every part of the bone marrow is representative of the other areas, with some remaining relatively normal. Blood disorders, such as leukaemia and myeloma (the 'haematological malignancies'), have a totally different pattern of behaviour from most 'solid' malignancies, though even in the latter, multiple primary tumours do occasionally occur in the same organ, including, for example, a rare form of lung cancer ('alveolar cell cancer'), in which several primary lung cancers develop, apparently much at the same time. Multiple primary site malignancy also occurs in the previously rare, but now all too common, Kaposi sarcoma so prevalent in young men with AIDS. One other rare skin condition, known as Gorlin's syndrome, is also characterised by multiple skin tumours of a very common type, which would normally occur as a single tumour.

Despite the single-site origin of most cancers, there is clearly an increased propensity, in many cases, for a second primary (not to be confused with tumour secondaries) to develop in other areas of similar tissue. This has an important bearing on the outcome and follow-up in patients with cancers of 'paired organs', such as the breast or testicle. There is no doubt that patients with breast cancer, though frequently successfully treated, do have a higher than expected incidence of a second primary tumour occurring in the opposite breast. The frequency with which this occurs has been variously recorded between five and twenty per cent. Likewise, in testicular tumours, second primary growths can occur in the opposite testis many years after unequivocal cure of the highly malignant tumour occurring at the initial site. Interestingly, one known causative feature of testicular cancer is the failure of testicular descent at or shortly after birth, and it is also clear that, whilst the poorly descended testicle is at greater risk of malignant change, a definite increased risk is noted in the testis which apparently developed and came down into the scrotal sac quite normally.

In some cancer patients, an obvious carcinogen may predispose them to more than one primary cancer developing. Perhaps the most tragic example of this occurs in patients who smoke heavily, develop an early and curable cancer of the larynx – often cured by radiotherapy without any loss of voice or serious side-effect – but then continue to smoke and develop a lung cancer a few years later, a disease with a far worse outlook and higher fatality rate than cancer of the larynx, and all too often incurable.

Cancers not only develop at a single site, but also result from malignant change within a single clone of cells. Our working hypothesis is that a single cell develops an irresistible pressure towards malignant change, presumably initiated by a genetic, environmental or other influence (or in most cases, of course, a combination of these) and develops into a malignant growth by continued cell division, producing progeny with the same characteristics and lack of cellular control. It is likely that a carcinogenic 'initiator' (the underlying or first event which destabilises the cell and renders it susceptible to cancer growth) is followed by one or more 'promoter' agents which produce further transient changes and which eventually cause the cancer to develop. We now know that several steps are required before a normal cell becomes a malignant one and that cell growth and division is profoundly influenced by the presence of critical genes which, as Professor Ponder of Cambridge has pointed out, conceptually fall into two groups: *oncogenes*, which drive the cell towards malignancy, and *suppressor* genes, which may mutate and result in a loss of normal regulatory or restraining function. It is often suggested that cellular oncogenes, when activated by carcinogens, initiate the events which lead to malignant transformation, and it may even be the case that certain viruses have incorporated these cellular genes into their own genetic templates, making them potential primers of malignant change occurring in mammalian or even human tissues at a later stage. Oncogenes may be very simply activated, becoming multiplied or amplified within the chromosome, to provide several copies, resulting in relatively rapid malignant development within the cell. An alternative method of growth might be the rearrangement of such genes between chromosomes, so that functional elements of the oncogene then disseminate still more rapidly within the cell and even beyond. With suppressor genes, on the whole more difficult to identify than oncogenes, a greater degree of abnormality – heredity of the abnormality from both parents, for example – may have to be present for the abnormal drive to be sufficient to initiate malignant change. This may turn out to be highly relevant in breast cancer, since the much-discussed, newly discovered BRCA-I gene on the 15q chromosome is thought most likely to be a suppressor gene acting in just this way. The central point is that loss of the tumour-suppressing activity of the critical gene, if present to a sufficient degree, may allow a tumour to develop. The presence and activity of tumour suppressor genes sits comfortably with traditional concepts of 'tumour surveillance', first postulated by Sir Peter Medawar and others forty years ago. He and other tumour biologists suggested that we might all be capable of producing potential cancers much of the time, but that some of us have a 'constant-alert' surveillance or scavenging cellular mechanism which recognises these potentially dangerous, early mutational changes and eliminates them before any real damage is done.

Good examples of the essential clonality – the initiation of cancer from a single cell – do occur in human cancers. In one study, for example, black women with an identifiable metabolic abnormality, known as G6PD deficiency, were carefully studied and their tumours characterised by chemical staining. Although normal tissue contains two different enzymes or chemical agents for G6PD, known as iso-enzymes, their tumour tissues were found to express only one or the other. The observation is, of course, consistent with the hypothesis that the tumour tissue arose from a single cell. In human myeloma, the abnormal cells are derived from characteristically large bone marrow plasma cells which would normally produce two types of protein material, kappa and lambda, whereas in myeloma and related disorders, it is easy to demonstrate that either the kappa or lambda protein chain is produced, but never both. All these observations point strongly towards the 'monoclonal' theory of cancer, as opposed to less dangerous types of cellular growth, for example in response to injury, in which cell regeneration is extremely important but well controlled ('polyclonal' growth).

The monoclonal nature of cancer has important diagnostic implications, since monoclonal antibodies can easily be prepared in laboratories, allowing recognition of the particular tissue of origin of certain human malignancies which were previously impossible to characterise. Since human tumours are often treated quite differently from each other, depending on the precise nature of the malignant tissue, these diagnostic refinements have important clinical consequences. Some types of tumour, for example, are so difficult to characterise by conventional microscope techniques that they are termed simply 'undifferentiated cancer'. In truth, they might have arisen from sites as different as the head and neck region, perhaps the nasopharynx, or the lymphatic tissue occupying lymph nodes (commonly termed 'glands'). Although sometimes indistinguishable by conventional examination of the biopsy slide under the microscope, the treatment of these conditions is so different that making the correct pathological diagnosis, often nowadays with the aid of monoclonal antibodies, is critical to accurate and successful treatment. For these reasons, cancer specialists seeing patients from other cancer centres will generally ask for the slides to be sent across, as well as the patient, so that these critical investigations can be made. In my own experience, this is often the most important single request a specialist can make, particularly when the patient comes from abroad where the diagnostic facilities may not be as good as those we now take for granted in large British hospitals.

In the future, it may be possible to use monoclonal antibodies therapeutically, as well as diagnostically. It is already possible to create an antibody to an apparently specific tumour antigen – the protein expressed solely by a tumour – and then to load it, for example, with a radioactive molecule so that the tumour, by picking up the specific monoclonal antibody, will also attract the radioactivity package towards itself, and thereby encourage it to self-destruct! This sounds wonderful, but there are many problems, including whether or not the tumour-related antigen really is specific, and whether the link between the antibody and the package of radioactivity can be sufficiently tight for cellular destruction to occur only on the surface of the malignant cell. Nevertheless, the idea of 'radio-immunotherapy' is an extremely attractive concept, possibly with a bright future ahead of it.

The other type of immunotherapy available for treatment of cancer is the non-specific 'stimulation' of the immune response that we probably all have in response to potential malignant change. Various agents have been used to supply this, notably BCG, the vaccine which is traditionally used to protect against the development of tuberculosis, and there is some evidence, particularly in the control of low-grade but widespread malignant growths covering the lining of the bladder, that such treatment can indeed be valuable. In the US, a large study of patients with cancer of the large bowel, treated with the non-specific immune stimulant levmisole in conjunction with chemotherapy, did seem to show a real advantage. Although this has now been accepted, at least in the USA, as offering the best treatment approach, the results are viewed with scepticism in the UK and other parts of Europe, as the probable benefits from this study could have resulted from the chemotherapy and not the immune stimulant drug.

Patterns of *spread* in human cancer

Despite the unchecked growth so typical of cancer at the cellular level, most types of malignant or 'neoplastic' growth display some degree of predictability in their evolution and pattern of spread. In general, there are three main patterns of behaviour, and each individual cancer type tends to behave in a characteristic way, though some malignant disorders are more predictable than others.

The major types of spread are by local extension, by lymphatic and lymph node involvement, and finally by blood-borne or haematogenous dissemination.

LOCAL EXTENSION

In this case, extension is by invasion of adjacent tissue, for example, invasion of a large primary breast cancer into skin, causing ulceration, or in lung cancer, local extension to an adjacent spinal vertebra, with erosion of the bone and potential damage to the spinal cord close by. The pattern of local invasiveness may also be affected by unwise surgery. For example, all surgical specialists know that the way to remove a primary testicular cancer is by a groin (inguinal) incision, with delivery of the testicle and attachments up through the groin, rather than by a direct surgical incision into the scrotum itself, because of the risk of 'seeding' the tumour or breaching the normal anatomic barrier that the fibrous capsule of the testicle provides. Cutting straight into a large cancer is extremely unwise and alway avoided – this is sometimes what the surgeon is rightly afraid of when he describes a cancer as inoperable, in other words, too large or attached to too many vital structures.

LYMPHATIC INVOLVEMENT

With lymphatic or lymph node spread, the tumour usually spreads initially to the local draining lymph nodes, though invasion to other lymph node sites, more distantly, also takes place. It is important to realise that most organs have a natural chain of draining lymph nodes which would normally remove excess tissue fluid, deal with local infectious processes and so on. In cancer, invasion of local lymph nodes is common and extremely important from the point of view of outcome (prognosis). For many tumours, the presence or absence of lymph node involvement is the most important single prognostic feature, defining with considerable accuracy which patients are likely to do well and which not. In breast cancer, for example, the presence of local lymph nodes in the axilla (the armpit area, i.e. the main site of drainage of lymph nodes relating to the breast) determines not only the likely outcome, but also predicts the degree of benefit from additional treatment, particularly chemotherapy. This point is discussed more fully in chapter 12. Breast cancer is particularly interesting in this respect, since there is a clear, quantitative relationship between the number of lymph nodes involved and the eventual, probable outcome. In head and neck cancer, the 'lymph node status', as it is termed, is again a highly predictive prognostic feature and may dictate whether or not a major operation to remove these glandular areas ('radical neck dissection') might have to be performed.

BLOOD-BORNE DISSEMINATION

Blood-borne or haematogenous metastasis is the most feared type of secondary spread in cancer and is not usually curable, though there are certain exceptions. Most specialists in the pathological and clinical care of cancer patients believe that tiny tumour deposits, possibly only single cells in the first instance, seed off from the main growth, setting down in various more or less hospitable sites within other parts of the body, and then capable of further growth at that secondary site. Certain organs, such as lung, bone and brain, seem much more likely to harbour these secondary deposits than, for example, heart, kidney or muscular areas of the body. Although no clear reason for this has ever been fully documented, it may well be that the degree of oxygenation of the tissues at these various sites has an important bearing. What we do know, however, is that certain types of cancer have particular patterns of spread with respect to the organs that are likely to be secondarily affected. Cancers of the head and neck areas, such as larynx, for example, tend, on the whole, to remain 'above the clavicles', so that local control of these tumours (including the important lymph node areas as well as the primary site) is usually tantamount to a cure. Breast cancer, on the other hand, has a particular predilection for spread to bone, brain, liver and lung, in addition to the lymph node drainage sites. Brain tumours are perhaps the most curious of all, since they may be highly malignant, with bizarre microscopic appearance and extreme difficulty in local control, particularly for the high-grade varieties, yet with almost no tendency whatsoever to metastasise to other parts of the body, and virtually no risk of lymph node invasion, even when the primary tumour cannot be surgically removed.

SPREAD ACROSS BODY CAVITIES

A fourth type of spread does occasionally occur, namely passage of tumour cells across a body cavity. Although unusual in most tumours, this is an extremely important mode of spread in patients with ovarian cancer, since the predominant pattern of tumour spread is within the abdomen, resulting from passage of tumour cells across from the initial pelvic site, within the abdominal cavity itself, and sometimes to the point of complete obliteration of this area, with cessation of vital functions (such as bowel activity) within it. Even though this type of spread may result in substantial uncontrolled growth and abdominal distension, these patients tend not to develop secondary tumours beyond the abdominal cavity, even where the tumour is hopelessly advanced and likely to be fatal within a short period.

In the particular group of lymphatic tumours termed 'lymphomas', spread to other lymph node areas is common, whereas direct invasion and haematogenous dissemination are less common than with 'solid' malignancies, despite the frequency of bone marrow involvement in many types of lymphoma This is also true, by and large, for leukaemia, in which the dangerous consequences are largely related to 'crowding out' of the normal bone marrow elements by the malignant process itself, leading to anaemia, infection as a result of poor function or insufficient numbers of white blood cells, and a tendency towards bleeding and easy bruising, as a result of loss of platelets, those tiny marrow cells which are largely responsible for the clotting mechanism.

COMBINATION OF TYPES OF SPREAD

Any or all of these processes can occur together, the clinical picture then depending, of course, on the speed at which these various events take place and the precise nature of the sites involved. For instance, in patients with secondary brain deposits, perhaps resulting from lung, breast or large bowel cancer, the clinical picture depends critically on the site of the secondary deposit, whether there is one such secondary or many, and also the speed at which the malignant dissemination has occurred. Since there are relatively 'silent' areas of the brain, i.e. areas with less critical functions than at other sites, primary or secondary tumours can grow in these areas with much less in the way of clinical manifestations than for other sites, such as the speech area, critically situated in the dominant hemisphere (normally the left side of the brain). A tumour appearing at this site would rapidly cause neurological changes. Surgical intervention is sometimes possible with secondary brain deposits, typically where there is only one tumour visualised, even by sophisticated scanning, and preferably in cases where it has developed at a less critical brain site, generally the lesser or non-dominant half (hemisphere) of the brain. This is because surgical excision will be less risky on the non-dominant side. Ideally it should be the only site of secondary spread, in a patient whose primary tumour was successfully treated some years before. In other cases (by far the majority, in fact), radiotherapy to the whole brain is a preferable form of treatment.

TUMOUR STAGING

The partially predictable nature of cancer dissemination has led to the concept of tumour staging, which is an important part of the initial investigation of many patients (though not all) with a proven malignant lesion. For a cancer specialist, it is particularly important to know the true extent of the possible spread of disease before embarking on treatment decisions, and separate tests may have to be performed to assess the extent of disease at the primary site (T), the extent, if any, of lymph node involvement (N) and the possible presence of more distant, blood-borne metastases (M). This TNM staging system is widely used, and specialists may speak, for example, of a T_3 N_1 M_0 laryngeal cancer, implying a primary tumour which is sufficiently locally advanced to have fixed the vocal cord, which is no longer mobile as it should be, together with relatively early lymph node invasion causing a palpable swelling in the neck, but not beyond a certain permissible size which would take the stage beyond the N_1 category. Finally, the M_0 means that there is no evidence of more extensive metastatic spread. For other tumour sites, such as breast, lung or oral cavity, the TNM system is based on different criteria. In the breast, for example, the T stage is dependent on a simple measurement of the primary tumour diameter (in centimetres), and in other sites, different staging criteria are more widely employed, for example the gynaecological cancers, in which either the FIGO (International Federation of Obstetrics and Gynaecology) or UICC (Union Internationale Contre le Cancer) give more consistent results. Brain tumours are again different, with a much greater emphasis on the *grade* of tumour, that is, its pathological appearance under the microscope, together with the degree to which the cells and tissue biopsy are regarded by the pathologist as departing from the normal appearance. In the commonest type of brain tumour, the group known as gliomas, four grades are internationally recognised by pathologists, with the lowest grade (grade 1) having a very good prognosis and many years (or more) of survival, whilst grade 4 lesions are extremely difficult to treat effectively, if at all. It is hardly surprising that all cancer specialists insist on a tissue biopsy wherever possible, in order to gain some idea of the proper treatment approach and the likely outcome.

One other important point about staging is that careful and consistent assessment of patients prior to treatment should then allow for a reasonably accurate comparison of results between different centres. How can you judge the claims of, say, a large American cancer centre that its new technique for brain tumours really is superior, without being sure that the patients apparently doing well are, in fact, closely comparable to those being treated at a less high-profile centre, say, in Britain or France? Although the best test of all is generally the prospectively randomised, controlled clinical trial (an area discussed in more detail in chapter 6), this approach is not always possible. The best we can do in such cases is to examine carefully the claims of the new treatment, with particular emphasis on assessing whether a large enough patient group has been treated by the new method for us to have real confidence in the results, and also whether or not they have been carefully assessed from the point of view of tumour-related prognostic factors before the treatment was begun.

Pathology of tumours

It is a common misconception that cancers are so bizarre in their appearance that the cells no longer bear any resemblance to the tissue of origin. Whilst this is occasionally true, it is the exception and not the rule. For solid tumours (a curious term, but one which serves well to distinguish most of the common cancers from the haematological malignancies such as leukaemia), the cancer is likely to be a 'carcinoma' or less commonly, a 'sarcoma'.

CARCINOMAS

The term 'carcinoma' implies a malignant tumour originating from an organ with a surface, either an external surface, such as skin, or an internal surface, such as the lining of the bronchial airways – giving rise to lung cancer – or of the lining of the upper or lower gastro-intestinal tract – giving rise, for example, to a carcinoma of the oesophagus or rectum. It may seem difficult to fit breast cancer into this category, but carcinomas of the breast and other glandular organs, such as the thyroid, stomach or pancreas, are essentially carcinomas originating at the surface, or 'epithelium', of the convoluted glandular structures within. If the tissue of origin is obviously glandular in this way, pathologists and clinicians would regard these as 'adenocarcinomas', whereas the more accessible carcinomas of skin, lower bowel and bronchus, together with the air and food passages that make up head and neck sites, are typically 'squamous carcinomas'. Put more accurately, the type of carcinoma is a reflection of the initial cell of origin, so adenocarcinomas arise from the cells of tissues in which glandular structures are a common feature, whereas squamous carcinomas arise from the surface or lining epithelium of cells which normally come into contact with the outside world – obvious in the case of skin, less so perhaps in the case of bronchus and rectum. One curious feature of lung cancer (still the commonest cause of malignancy, particularly in males, in the Western world) is that the normal lining of the bronchus is not with squamous cell epithelium at all; it is the prolonged exposure to cigarette smoke which alters the cells from their normal ('columnar') form into squamous cells, a term known as squamous metaplasia, and, more importantly, a change which may then progress further toward malignancy.

SARCOMAS

Sarcomas are primary cancer growths of soft tissue and occasionally bone, and generally regarded as highly malignant in their pattern of behaviour. These tumours arise within muscle, bone or joint spaces and are difficult to characterise microscopically. Each is known by a separate label – leiomyosarcoma, in the case of a smooth muscle primary, such as the uterus or womb (as distinct from a uterine adenocarcinoma, much more common, in which the lining cells of the uterus become malignant) or rhabdomyosarcoma in the case of a malignant tumour of 'striped' muscle, i.e. one under voluntary active control, for instance the muscles of locomotion within the thigh or arm. These are much less common tumours than the carcinomas and they behave in a different way. Unlike the majority of cancers, which occur predominantly (but not exclusively) in older age groups, the sarcomas which arise as primary bone tumours tend to occur in the adolescent age group. One of the greatest advances in cancer treatment during recent years is the recognition that most young people affected by this disorder can be adequately treated by local surgical removal of the offending part of bone, together with chemotherapy and sometimes radiation therapy, without the need for amputation as was the case until about twenty years ago. This is discussed in chapter 22.

TUMOUR NECROSIS

Although the growth of cancer cells was previously described as being typically uncontrolled and unchecked, this is not by any means the whole story. As cancers become larger, they begin to outstrip their blood supply and their innermost, least well-oxygenated cells typically begin to slow down or may even lose their viability altogether. This is often called tumour necrosis, and may result in a visible change, for example on a chest X-ray, in which a solid growth may visibly alter in appearance to what looks like a cyst or abscess, but in truth is the poorly oxygenated, poorly nourished interior of the tumour which is undergoing breakdown or tissue necrosis. Unfortunately, the rim or edge will still retain its previous capability, so tumour necrosis is never followed by a spontaneous cure. There is considerable diversity in the rate of growth of tumours, some growing rather slowly, often accompanied by tumour cell necrosis and slow local progression, while others have a much more rapid tempo altogether, often with early dissemination to other organs. Two major types of lung cancer illustrate this point well. Firstly, in the typical squamous cell carcinoma of the lung or bronchus, tumour growth is often relatively slow, and the specialist may, for various reasons, decide to watch and wait rather than immediately opt for active treatment in every individual case; however, the 'small-cell' type of lung cancer, the disease most characteristically associated with cigarette smoking, is extremely virulent and rapid in its evolution, with very early dissemination to secondary sites and a very poor overall prognosis, despite initial responsiveness to chemotherapy. One major cancer site, two separate types of pathology, two completely different types of malignant behaviour, and, as a result, requiring quite different treatment.

CANCER AND THE CELL CYCLE

On the whole, cancer cells do divide more rapidly than tumour tissue, often to a remarkable degree. The 'doubling time' (the rate at which a tumour might be expected to double its volume, all other things being equal) can be as little as a few days, though this is much more true in the very earliest, microscopic, stages of a tumour's development rather than later on, where the tumour is easily visible on a chest X-ray or even by touch, at which point it has usually slowed down considerably. Each cell, however, has to be produced from a malignant precursor, passing through the various stages of the cell cycle which are so critical for division. After each cell division, the cell enters a growth phase (G_1), though there may be a period of quiescence (G_0), during which it has little if any potential for growth or malignant change. G_1 is followed by the phase of DNA synthesis, the S phase, in which the chromosomal material within the nucleus of the cell, and of course the DNA contained within it, is doubled in preparation for cell division at a later stage. First it has to pass through a further growth phase (G_2), prior to the active phase of cell division, *mitosis*, in which at last the pairs of chromosomes separate and the cell divides, with both progeny capable of further malignant growth and subsequent cell division. The key difference between cancer and normal cells is that the normal controlling mechanisms of the cell cycle have been lost, and the cell progeny continue to grow and divide until checked by treatment – either surgical removal or an effective method of inhibiting growth, generally by radiotherapy, hormone treatment or chemotherapy. Spontaneous regressions of cancer are extremely rare. Although well documented in certain childhood tumours, a true spontaneous regression, without treatment of any kind, does not occur with a true cancer. Most cases of apparent spontaneous recovery from cancer are either treatment related or incorrectly diagnosed as cancer in the first place.

It is important to realise that cancers are only truly detectable towards the end of their biological lives. Early phases of cell doubling following the mutational change in response to the initiation/promotion-induced cellular alterations (themselves a response to carcinogenic, genetic or combined influences) are generally undetectable. The only exception to this is in the case of tumours which elaborate a cell marker, generally a protein or other substance which is specific to the tumour and manufactured by it, secreted into the bloodstream, and which can then be detected, generally by sensitive radio-immunoassay or other tests. A good example is in testicular tumours, many of which elaborate two well-recognised marker substances – AFP (alpha feto-protein) and beta HCG (human chorionic gonadotrophin) – each of which can be assayed in the blood and may well be detectable at abnormally high levels after apparently successful treatment of the primary tumour, at a time when there is no other evidence of the reappearance of the tumour. In these exceptional circumstances, treatment of the recurrence can properly commence whilst the tumour burden is relatively modest, without waiting for other evidence of failure of the initial therapeutic approach.

Testicular tumours of this kind are an ideal clinical example, since not only is the height of the abnormal marker a clear reflection of the degree of relapse, but also the marker itself can be measured reliably, and we have a highly effective means of chemotherapeutic treatment of indivi-duals who relapse, regardless of where in the body that relapse might be. In other tumours, we are far less fortunate, since they either fail to produce a recognisable marker, or, as in the case of primary liver cancer, which may also secrete AFP, no satisfactory treatment exists, apart from surgery, for the initial primary tumour.

It is clear that some apparently normal subjects (not yet patients, but destined to become them) have a high susceptibility to certain types of cancer, a point discussed in chapter 2. Little is known of the cellular regulating mechanisms which prevent patients who have a strong genetic predisposition from developing their cancer(s) earlier in life. Think, for example, of the extraordinary phenomenon of colo-rectal (large bowel) cancer, a common condition with over 28,000 new cases a year in the United Kingdom, which can generally be cured by surgery if the tumour is detected early enough, without evidence of spread. Scientists have now located the gene which causes bowel cancer, situated on the second main chromosome (out of twenty-three human pairs), following painstaking work on two substantial families with a history of the disease. The work required collaboration between three major research groups in the United States and Finland, and it is now estimated that the defective gene is carried by one in every 200 people in the Western population, or viewed from a different perspective, up to 250,000 people in Britain alone, making this the most common inherited disorder of all. Within the next few years, this should allow testing of high-risk families on a very large scale, with the prospect either of careful regular screening for patients carrying the gene but without evidence of the disease, or possibly early surgery in selected cases. Now that we have relatively straightforward means of direct examination of the whole large bowel using fibre-optic methods (colonoscopy), the careful study of such potential patients is technically possible. The difficulty will be in assessing the relative costs and benefits of such an enormous task.

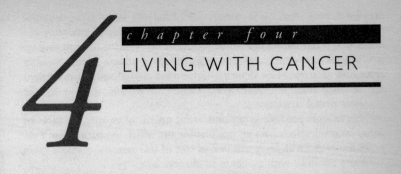

chapter four

LIVING WITH CANCER

Symptoms

Since cancer can arise from such a wide variety of sites and develop with so many differing patterns of spread, there are no clear-cut symptoms which unequivocally give the game away. In this respect, cancer is unlike many, more specific, non-malignant ailments such as heart disease, in which chest pain, shortness of breath, exercise limitation and a few other symptoms are so often present. The arthritic diseases, characterised by joint pain and stiffness, are another good example. With cancer, the precise nature of the symptoms depends not only on the primary site, but specifically where within the offending organ the tumour is located, the rate of development, and also whether or not symptoms of secondary spread are already present. Occasionally, the symptoms and physical signs of secondary spread occur even before the primary site has declared itself, and from time to time, the initial primary, from which all else has developed, never becomes apparent. This clearly poses particular difficulties both for the patient and the doctor, and these difficult cases are dealt with separately in chapter 22.

Many primary tumours cause local swelling if they arise at a visible or accessible part of the body, such as skin, breast, testicle or oral cavity. A typical tumour swelling is initially painless, though ulceration (skin breakdown) can occur, which may sometimes be painful. Some patients seek medical advice early, when there is a small swelling, and are sometimes wrongly reassured, particularly if the enlargement is a glandular one, for example in the neck. It is easy for specialists to decry the lack of vigilance of general practitioners who may disregard such early warning signs, yet the truth is that the probable cause of the glandular neck swelling is much more likely to be a non-malignant problem than cancer – simple viral illnesses, infectious mononucleosis (glandular fever) and so on. In the mouth, a non-healing ulcer or sore on the tongue may mistakenly be regarded as a simple ulcer, possibly secondary to a traumatic denture, rather than recognised as a malignant lesion; such cases are often later referred to an oral surgeon by the patient's dental practitioner.

Skin cancers produce symptoms early, unless, of course, the ulcer or other lesion develops over an inaccessible site which the patient can't see – on the back or under a nail bed of one of the toes, for example. Skin tumours are dealt with in detail in chapter 18.

With lung cancer, the symptoms may be particularly difficult for the patient and doctor to evaluate, since many smokers have chronic bronchitic complaints, with coughing, wheezing, shortness of breath and chest pain as relatively common complaints that they have become used to. It can be extremely difficult to recognise that the nature of the symptoms has changed, unless a specific complaint, such as haemoptysis (coughing up blood), has developed, which then may alert the general practitioner to ask for a chest X-ray or a referral to a specialist. Curiously, one early feature which many chest physicians have noted is the frequency with which such patients give up smoking, apparently quite easily in many cases, despite a lifetime punctuated with multiple, half-hearted or unsuccessful attempts whilst the patient was still relatively fit. It happens so frequently that one can't help wondering whether there is either some innate abhorrence of cigarettes once the lung cancer has taken root, or, perhaps more realistically, a recognition by the patient that this particular group of symptoms is more serious than before, even though this change in symptomatology may not be transmitted to the physician.

TRAUMA AND CANCER

Other groups of symptoms are discussed in relation to the specific tumour sites in chapters 11–22, but one general point worth mentioning is the vexed relationship between trauma and cancer development. Patients frequently report a knock or injury during the month or two preceding the development of what turns out to be a cancer and may well associate the two. The conventional medical view is that there is no known relationship between traumatic injury of this type and the development of cancer, and, in any event, it would be quite outside the normal understood concept (and time relations) of cancer development. Many patients seem to feel more satisfied if they can pin the development of cancer on a specific episode, as if this 'understanding' somehow makes the disease more palatable and brings some sense into what is otherwise a completely baffling situation. The commonest tumours in which one hears a history of this kind are breast, testis and the much less common primary bone tumours of late childhood and adolescence, in which the history of a sporting or other type of trauma is frequent. The truth of the matter is probably that these events are well remembered and relatively common in this physically active phase of life. What also might be true, however, is that a significant traumatic injury could perhaps cause local tissue swelling and internal bruising around the tumour, accentuating the swelling which, up until that point, may have been extremely subtle and hard to detect. The same is probably true for testicular tumours, predominantly diseases of younger men, and surprisingly hard to detect, since enlargement of the testicle beyond its normal size is generally painless and often difficult to recognise in its early stages. In short, traumatic injury and the development of cancer are thought to be unrelated.

Making the diagnosis

BIOPSIES

Some form of biopsy is all important and will almost invariably need to be performed, since it is imperative to make a firm and unequivocal diagnosis of cancer, if the patient really has it, and to then go further and gain as much information about the type of cancer as possible. Even in elderly, infirm patients, it can be a serious mistake to treat 'on spec' without a biopsy, since sooner or later, it may become more difficult to decide whether to proceed to additional treatment, if a watertight diagnosis has not been established.

The best and most secure form of biopsy is one which gives the pathologist (i.e. the non-clinical specialist who peers down the microscope and uses a variety of staining and other techniques on thin microscope slide sections of tumour prepared from the original block of tissue) as much material as required to make a complete diagnosis. Many large departments will use this tissue not only for diagnosing the individual patient, but for research as well, and all are required by law to retain the original tumour block, generally embedded in paraffin wax, for many years. In doubtful cases, where the diagnosis can be extremely difficult, slides can easily be sent from one centre to another, or even across to other parts of the world for further opinions. The critical role of the tumour biopsy in diagnosis was recently highlighted by the tragic events at the Birmingham Bone Tumour Centre, where it became apparent that incorrect diagnoses had been made over a number of years, leading, sadly, to a number of cases in which inappropriate treatment, even including amputation, might have been given. All surgical teams know that this small surgical operation is of critical value, particularly where the biopsy is the first that has been taken in the illness. There may be more to follow, if, for example, a recurrence of the disease is suspected at a later date.

It may be sufficient for the patient to undergo a fine needle biopsy, usually providing sufficient material for a specialised pathologist, known as a cytologist, to obtain a semi-solid smear specimen, which is then fixed onto the microscope slide and rapidly interpreted, often within a day or two. Whilst this does not yield as much material as the formal histopathological specimen from a scalp biopsy, it is usually quite sufficient to make a diagnosis of cancer with as minimal trauma to the patient as possible, allowing a cool and dispassionate decision with regard to treatment, coupled, of course, with a discussion with the patient in the light of a firmly established diagnosis. Fine needle aspiration is generally performed under a simple local anaesthetic as an out-patient procedure, whereas a formal biopsy, using a surgical technique and leaving a one- or two-centimetre scar, may occasionally require a general anaesthetic. In the case of skin tumours, it is often possible to remove, or excise, these completely, thus gaining both the diagnosis and, in many cases, adequate therapy at the same time.

OTHER MEANS OF DIAGNOSIS

In patients with lung cancer who are producing sputum from the chest, this can be sent for analysis, searching for any malignant cells which might be present, again giving a firm diagnosis without the need for further biopsy. In this respect, lung cancer may be similar to cancer of the cervix, in which the same sort of cytology technique, this time using a wooden spatula to gain material directly from the cervix, has been highly successful in yielding a diagnosis not only of probable cancer, but also, in a larger proportion of cases, varying degrees of pre-cancerous change (see chapter 14). Generally speaking, the pathologist will report certain technical details about the cancer, once the diagnosis has been established, and many clinicians regard the written pathological diagnostic report as perhaps the most important single investigation performed during the patient's illness. The pathologist's report of cancer will be based on the appearance of the cells, their relationship to each other, the degree to which they no longer resemble the cells from a normal slide of that type of tissue, and also the rate at which cells are actively dividing (the mitotic rate), which, in cancer, is generally higher than normal. Equally important is the observation of tumour invasiveness, with, typically, an identifiable area in which the deep layer of the tissue of origin (often termed the 'basement membrane') is clearly breached by the ingrowing tumour. This invasiveness is rightly regarded as one of the cardinal pathological features of cancer.

For all the reasons discussed in chapter 3, it is important at this stage to consider whether further information is required about the tumour before making a decision with regard to treatment. In many cases, this will involve further blood tests, X-rays, ultrasound scanning and/or isotope scans. What might be necessary for one type of tumour could be completely inappropriate in another; for example, in a small primary skin tumour of the commonest type seen in the UK, no staging investigations are required at all, whereas in patients with Hodgkin's disease, one of the group of lymphomas, full scanning is advisable, since a patient with an enlarged gland or lymph node in the neck may have occult (but radiologically detectable) disease in the central part of the chest or even within the abdomen. The commonest blood tests requested by the specialist are likely to be a full blood count, in order to check that the patient is neither anaemic nor lacking in other important blood elements, and simple blood analyses of liver and renal (kidney) function. In many centres, it is common in patients with breast cancer for the physician to request a bone scan, using a very small dose of radioactive isotope as a tracer, in order to delineate the bones and make certain that there is no sign of early spread to this site; though, in truth, the rate of detection by this method is not high, and fewer and fewer departments are performing this routinely, since the cost benefit return is poor.

RADIOLOGY AND SCANNING

The dramatic revolution in diagnostic radiology over the past twenty years has enormously benefited cancer patients. Whereas we used to be limited to relatively simple X-rays or ultrasound scans, we now have wonderfully sophisticated computer tomography (CT) and magnetic resonance imaging (MRI), both of which give remarkably accurate visualisation of the internal structure of various parts of the body. CT scanning is excellent for the chest, particularly since small secondary tumour nodules in the lungs may be visualised by this technique in cases where a simple chest X-ray could appear normal. In other parts of the body, including brain, spinal cord and pelvis, the MRI scan is likely to be superior, particularly since it can take images in virtually any plane (unlike CT scanning), and can be repeated more frequently (since it involves no radiation exposure) in order to monitor progress without any danger to the patient. Repeat CT or MRI scanning often represent the best possible means of monitoring or following up a patient's progress after treatment has been given; these scans are as useful in this respect as they are for the original diagnosis and staging of the untreated tumour.

Ultrasound scanning, though less glamorous perhaps than CT or MRI, has the advantage that it is inexpensive, easy to perform, easily repeatable and without any known dangers. It is excellent for gaining information about the internal anatomy of the abdomen and pelvis, and in particular is often used to assess whether or not the liver is involved in the cancer process. Recently, internal probes have been introduced, both for ultrasound and other types of scanning, which allow more direct and accurate inspection of the pelvis, via the vaginal or rectal routes. This can give excellent imaging of, for example, the prostate gland sitting just beneath the bladder (often involved in cancer in elderly men) and the cervix and upper pelvic organs in women.

DECIDING ON TREATMENT

Once these investigations have been completed, together with tumour markers (if appropriate), special X-rays and, if necessary, careful direct inspection by fibre-optic endoscopic procedures (using flexible internal telescopes), the specialist is generally in a position to make a decision with regard to treatment. The whole aim of this lengthy and frustrating preliminary exercise is to provide sufficient information for a properly informed judgement to be made. The tests may influence the oncologist towards or away from surgery, for example, or may even point to a 'watch and wait' policy rather than active treatment. It is far better to take a few extra days to get this crucial information, than to rush into an inappropriate form of treatment.

When the treatment discussion takes place, the patient should feel free to ask any questions and should not hesitate to use this opportunity, since many consultants, myself included, feel that the first one or two consultations with a patient are likely to be both the most important and, in all probability, the most lengthy. This may well be the best opportunity the patient has for clarification of all the issues that are bothering him or her. A good doctor should always try and avoid appearing rushed; indeed, one of the most important skills is to converse with the patient in such a way that he or she feels comfortable, relaxed and, preferably, that there is no one else in the world the doctor would sooner be with at that moment! It is true that most doctors are busy and overworked, but most, too, are sensitive human beings who enjoy their work and realise that time spent talking at this early stage is a good investment, from everybody's point of view, for the future. I often remind medical students that the patients' lives continue outside the consulting room and that they have you for just a brief moment, so try and make it easy for them to use that time in the best possible way.

They should also be encouraged to bring a friend or family member with them for these important discussions – this will help the doctor and patient's mutual understanding, since patients often have great difficulty coping with their anxieties, fears and uncertainties, all of which make it more difficult for the doctor's information to be properly perceived and registered.

A tape recorder can be helpful as well, though many doctors (myself included) find it slightly unnerving. The only real problem I have with family members sitting in on the discussion is when they start to ask the questions which *they* want answered, without the patient voicing them him- or herself. Not a problem, perhaps, if it's a straighforward point, such as, 'How many courses of chemotherapy did you say he would probably need, doctor?', but what if the wife, sister, friend asks, 'Just how long will he have, doctor?' This isn't so easy. I'm all for honesty in these matters, but how does the poor doctor know whether this weighty question is one which the patient wants answered? At the end of the day, my prime responsibility is to the patient, not the family member, and if there is ever any question of conflict between them, I have to be on the patient's side, even if I think, in some cases, the family are being more rational. In the example just noted, I don't on the whole feel I can answer such a question, or even attempt to, unless it's the patient who makes it clear he or she wishes to know; so I would have to turn to them, and ask as gently as I could whether or not that was a question they wanted answered. Even that, of course, is an intrusion! It puts the patient on the spot in a way they might well have preferred to avoid. The point I'm trying to make is that, in my view, it's not for the family and friends to put questions of that kind at all, unless there's been a previous agreement between the patient and themselves. I think patients have a right to ask questions, or not, as they see fit, and have those questions honestly dealt with by the doctor. It's the role of the companion to support, remind the patient of particular points they had previously said they wanted to cover, perhaps to take them for a coffee afterwards, and then to get them home.

One important distinction which the doctor needs to have in mind at the early treatment stage is whether or not he or she is aiming for cure or not. This, of course, will depend on the nature of the problem and the patient's ability to withstand a treatment programme that necessarily would be much more intensive and taxing if cure was the aim – a radical treatment. In cases where the cancer is clearly not curable (and most patients who have established secondary deposits would fall into this category), it is fruitless, pointless, ill-judged and a waste of everyone's time and energy for such intensive treatment to be recommended. The appropriate form of treatment would be palliative, that is, a less ambitious programme directed towards control of symptoms. Surprisingly, perhaps, some patients with cancer have no symptoms at all. If the patient clearly cannot be cured and has no symptoms, many a specialist would (in my view, rightly) recommend a programme of careful follow-up, but not necessarily press treatment at this initial stage.

At the other extreme, in curable disorders in fit, young patients, treatment might have to be very intensive indeed, and possibly prolonged over a year or so for maximum benefit and likelihood of cure. In all cases, the patient should ideally come away from the initial consultation(s) with a clear understanding of what the doctor has said, why it was said, what the alternatives might be and the likely time scale of the proposed treatment. Although many patients are still fully prepared to place themselves in the doctor's hands, in the traditional and flattering way, many more aren't these days! Doctors have had to get used to these more detailed discussions, whether they like or not – and most realise that they do, in fact, prefer it, because it allows a true partnership to develop between doctor and patient, rather than, as in the time-honoured way, the patient being little more than a passive recipient of the medical advice.

Follow-up appointments will be recommended by the doctor for a whole variety of reasons. First of all, of course, the doctor will need to see how the patient is getting on, in order to determine whether or not there has been a response to treatment and whether the programme needs to be modified in any way. Secondly, it may be necessary to repeat some of the more detailed or complicated parts of the discussion. Thirdly, we often have students with us who need to see as many patients as possible during their training years – this may well apply to postgraduate as well as undergraduate students. Finally, it does also help the doctor enormously to continue seeing patients well after the treatment is completed, not only for strictly medical reasons, but because most doctors have a genuine human interest in the patient's life, and there is, of course, a good deal of professional pride and gratification following patients over a long period. Most cancer patients will be followed up at regular intervals, gradually lessening in frequency, from diagnosis until either death or a minimum of five years. This is generally not necessary, though, for tumours which are usually easily curable, such as small skin tumours.

Most patients realise that, for the first few years at least, there is considerable uncertainty as to whether they are genuinely cured. Fortunately, most don't dwell on it; indeed, I often feel that the ability to cast the uncertainty to one side is a remarkable attribute that many patients display to a most impressive degree. One can't of course change one's personality, but too much broody introspection on the part of the patient is not in my view likely to be all that helpful, though the doctor must of course support the patient's fears and anxieties, which are likely to be expressed to their greatest degree during the first few months after treatment has been completed. Many patients, in fact, find that this is the most difficult time of all. Up to that point, they will have been 'centre stage', so to speak, and have regularly been coming to the hospital, with that powerful support of the next treatment or follow-up visit only a few weeks away. To be suddenly cast adrift at the end of it all and told that they don't need to return for two or three months can be extremely alarming, and the transformation from patient back to normal human being needs to be handled with great skill, not only by the specialist but by the patient's general practitioner as well. It is all too easy for doctors to forget that patients with cancer are often facing the greatest crisis of their lives and may need constant support and time to discuss their fears. It can be difficult to provide the reassurance that many wish for, though a sympathetic ear must always be available. Many of the best cancer departments operate an 'open-door' policy, so that patients needing reassurance or a further discussion should feel able to phone the department and come within a very few days, regardless of the date of their next follow-up appointment.

In recent years, there has been an increasing discussion of patient participation in the choice of treatment, a trend which I strongly support. Clearly, patients can share in the decision-making only if they are well informed about the options, but there can be drawbacks too. As a recent, independent report for doctors pointed out, 'One fear is that exploring treatment options may confront the patient with the advanced nature of his or her cancer, and thus induce despair.' Nonetheless, the majority of patients receiving active treatment do wish to have as much information as possible. Interestingly enough, there are specific groups who appear to want more information, including, in general, younger and better educated patients, whereas older patients, particularly men, often seem to prefer to leave more of the decisions to their carers.

Sharing responsibility for treatment decisions does, however, appear to have psychological benefits for many. For example, in the reduction of anxiety and depression pre- and post-operatively in patients with breast cancer, the adequacy of information supplied by the medical team seems to be the main factor in reducing long-term psychological consequences of the illness and its treatment. In all these discussions, both initial and follow-up, it is extremely important to avoid the use of medical jargon, a device which too many doctors hide behind. You must somehow find the right phrases, the right words, steering a path between the smoke-screen of medical terminology and unacceptable condescension. We know that the way that information is presented certainly affects patients' choices about treatment options, so to help the patient achieve a really balanced view, information may have to be presented by the doctor in a variety of ways, or repeatedly over two or three sessions. This is particularly the case when treatment involves a number of steps, possibly including referral to a second specialist or when the doctor needs to introduce the concept of a clinical trial because of uncertainty as to the best way forward. This is discussed in more detail in chapter 6.

Living with uncertainty

We often read a newspaper headline 'TV soap star cured of cancer', yet halfway down the page, it becomes clear that treatment was only completed last week! Such over-simplification, to the point of trivialising the problem and insulting the readers' intelligence, does no good to any of us, least of all the TV soap star. The truth, of course, is that years have to elapse before one can state with any certainty that a patient might genuinely be cured; the length of time depends on the nature of the cancer and the statistical probability of relapse at specific time intervals after the initial treatment.

There are some cancers which are so rapidly evolving, so lethal if untreated, that a clear passage of two years after treatment, without evidence of relapse, is all that is necessary for the patient to be declared cured, genuinely cured. For small cell lung cancer, for instance, and most types of testicular cancer, a clean bill of health during the two-year period, without any evidence of relapse or further medical problems, does usually mean just that. With breast cancer, on the other hand, with a quite different behaviour and natural history, two years is far too short an interval; indeed, even the traditionally used five-year point is insufficient, since relapses can occur even at ten years and beyond. For the doctor, this makes breast cancer the most challenging but frustrating of cancers to treat, since genuine advances in treatment methods will inevitably take many years of painstaking clinical research to measure and assess. It's important never to confuse novelty with progress.

The statistical chances of a patient relapsing or developing evidence of secondary cancers does, of course, have a bearing on the likely programme of follow-up care. For example, in cancers of the head and neck area, such as larynx, tongue, pharynx, etc., the overwhelming probability is that relapse will occur, if it is going to happen at all, within the first three years of initial treatment. For this reason, many specialists recommend a routine pattern of follow-up care, with monthly hospital visits for examination during the first year of follow-up, every two months during the second and every three months during the third, matching the possibility of failure of treatment to its statistical probability over that first three-year period. Likewise, many specialists ask breast-cancer patients to return only every six months or so after the five-year point has been reached.

Doctors do have to be careful though – I remember one patient who had been concerned about her five-year survival chances, coming back at the five-year point amazed that she was still alive at all and (to my shame, since it was I who told her in the first place) having gained no real understanding that a seventy per cent chance of remaining alive and well at five years implied that there was a very good chance of continuing healthy and free of disease even well beyond that time. Repetition of information, advice or even instructions, whilst often so irritating in the domestic setting, can be of the greatest importance as part of the professional consultation.

It is uncertainty about relapse, failure of treatment and ultimately death from cancer which represent the patient's greatest fears. Repeat follow-up visits may do much to alleviate this distress, and the patient of course, will generally (but not always) derive considerable satisfaction from the knowledge that the specialist is both competent and accessible. Many find it extremely valuable to meet other patients who have suffered in the same way, and mutual self-help groups are now very much part of the scene, some hospital based and some responding to a patient's preference to meet like-minded others as far away from the hospital setting as possible.

Most large cancer centres also have counsellors, sometimes for specific complaints such as breast, lung or gynaecological cancer. In my own department, we have full-time counsellors who are present within the out-patient department itself, and are prepared to see patients, relatives and staff. This seems to me as good a place as any to express my warm admiration, appreciation and personal thanks to them, though I must also state that, in my view, the availability of skilled counsellors does not in any way absolve the doctor from a most important counselling and advisory role. It is quite wrong for doctors to feel that they can properly shift this burden to others, since there are inevitably many questions which only a doctor can answer. Which doctor would wish to become simply a mechanistic purveyor of the various available treatments, without the more discursive and pastoral elements of doctoring that should go with it?

COPING WITH RELAPSE

One of the most difficult and upsetting parts of cancer medicine concerns the proper physical and psychological management of the patient who has relapsed at a distant (secondary) site, for the first time after an apparently successful initial treatment, and who has thus gone from being a potentially cured patient to one in whom cure is almost certainly no longer possible – and perhaps with a relatively limited life span. It seems to me that a profoundly important point of inflection has been reached, often all in a moment, and for the most part this situation has become apparent only to the doctor, not the patient. It may take far more time than is available at that single consultation for the doctor to take a view as to the best way forward, and in particular, the best way of imparting this knowledge to the patient, if indeed this is done at all. I don't believe that there are obvious rules about this, though some may argue that, in such situations, the doctor has no right at all to withhold such information; the very least he or she should do is tell the patient the truth. Once again, however, whilst applauding this as a general view and for the most part acting on it, I do feel that there are sometimes exceptions. Many elderly patients have no great hopes for life expectancy anyway, and have already set their affairs in order; the older generation is, in my view, not quite as demanding of 'absolute information' at all times as those of us who are younger, possibly better educated, and members of different social cultures in which as much information as possible is expected under all circumstances. Many elderly patients might be suffering from other disorders, such as heart disease, which are likely to cause an earlier death than, say, a slow-growing secondary deposit from breast cancer. What is important, however, is to think carefully about the options for palliative treatment at this point and to give the best care, regardless of whether or not it is likely to lead to a cure.

Lifestyle and cancer

When cancer has been detected and treated, and a patient returned (hopefully) to a relatively normal life, what advice should be given?

'How should I conduct myself now doctor?' was the way one, highly respectable, retired army colonel with lung cancer put it to me once. 'Should it be don't smoke, don't drink, live clean?' was his second question, and we both smiled – me out of gratitude to him for taking the lead.

He was surprised when I told him I didn't altogether agree with this strict regime. Not smoking, of course, is the best possible recommendation one could give to people anxious to avoid getting cancer in the first place, but there is no terribly convincing evidence that, once the cancer has developed, stopping smoking is likely to be a key part of the patient's recovery though it's certainly important to discontinue, if possible, during a course of radiotherapy. Frankly, if the lung cancer is clearly incurable, as is so often the case, it will lead to the patient's early death within, say, three years, regardless of whether he or she smokes or not. Although many patients in this situation have stopped smoking already, it would be absurd and cruel to point out that they have done it far too late. I'm not sure that patients who are still smoking, who have enough on their plate coping with uncertainty, investigation, treatment and so on, should necessarily have to cope with what would inevitably be another major pressure. Some of my colleagues may be aghast at this cavalier view, but many patients regard their cigarette, like their cup of tea or coffee, as a welcome means of punctuating the day. There is, however, good evidence that patients with cancers of the head and neck who stop smoking and drinking during treatment (such patients often are rather heavy smokers and fond of alcohol too) tolerate the treatment better and have a better prognosis (outlook) in the long run. The more important point, however, is that patients who have a *curable* cancer, even one which is likely to have been cigarette-induced, most certainly should be advised to stop smoking as soon as possible. Like all cancer specialists, I have seen too many tragic cases of patients cured of one cancer going on to develop a second and fatal primary cancer through continued cigarette smoking.

There is some important evidence about alcohol as well. Clearly it plays a part in the development of certain tumours, notably the primary head and neck cancers mentioned above (particularly those of the oral cavity) and also in the development of primary liver cancer, which is a rather uncommon tumour in the Western world, but with a very high prevalence in the Middle and Far East. However, I don't think it's necessary to insist that all cured cancer patients should give up alcohol entirely, though it's certainly best to be moderate – and in any event, for general health reasons, alcohol moderation is clearly wise. Both the Royal College of General Practitioners and Royal College of Psychiatrists recognise alcohol-related problems as being far more common than is normally accepted, and current guidelines for alcohol intake are considerably lower than what was traditionally viewed as acceptable – twenty-one units per week for men, fourteen units per week for women. A unit of alcohol is the equivalent of half a pint of beer, a glass of wine, or a single measure of spirits. I don't personally feel that cancer patients (or ex-patients) need to be warned to reduce their alcohol intake below these levels, although those with a past history of alcohol-induced cancer may, in my experience, find it easier to give it up altogether.

As for sex, there is no need to apply any restrictions whatever. Many will find, of course, that the diagnosis of cancer, and its treatment, lead to loss of libido in the short term, and patients may need to be warned about this and to be reassured that it is both commonplace and generally short-lived. Others will find cancer such a powerful emotional experience that it changes all aspects of their lives, including perhaps their sexuality, for months, years or even permanently. While a diagnosis of cancer in one partner may well bring a couple closer together, in others it may do the reverse, particularly, one presumes, if the partnership or marriage was shaky in the first place. What is really important, however, is that husbands, wives and partners should all be aware of their critically important supportive role and be prepared to take the emotional flak which will inevitably come their way. The rewards follow later. Some may even need reminding that cancer is not infectious and that human warmth, understanding and touch are more important than ever. True recovery takes more than the return of physical health and functioning; I can't avoid repeating the cliché that emotional scars take far longer to heal.

As far as the psychological aspects of supportive care are concerned, I felt on reflection that this was a wide enough subject to deserve a chapter of its own. Talking to so many patients about these issues over many years it struck me that the most concise way of dealing with this – at least the practical issues raised, if not the philosophical, cultural and (dare I say it) existential – would be to tackle this in question-and-answer format (chapter 25, page 269).

There is a host of organisations, some national, others on a smaller scale, designed to support and benefit patients (and their families) with cancer. A full list is provided at the end of this book.

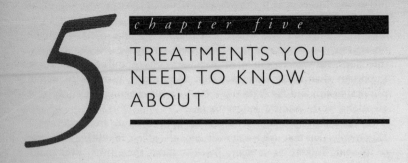

chapter five

TREATMENTS YOU NEED TO KNOW ABOUT

Introduction

Cancer medicine is one of the most rapidly moving of all medical specialities, both in the fields of science and understanding, and also treatment. Although there is evidence that cancer was recognised as a specific group of diseases and treated by primitive surgical methods even before the Christian era, the tentative beginnings of modern cancer techniques had to await the end of the nineteenth century for the development of safer surgical techniques and the discovery, almost simultaneously, of natural radioactivity by the Curies and artificial X-ray production by Röntgen. Radiation and surgery were effectively the only means of treatment during the early part of this century, but in the 1940s, two remarkable therapeutic steps were made. First, in 1941, Charles Huggins published his findings on a totally new hormone treatment, generally by means of bilateral orchidectomy (castration) in patients with advanced prostate cancer, demonstrating for the first time that responses could occur when no further conventional treatment was possible. And secondly, a series of anti-cancer chemotherapy agents was discovered and developed, notably nitrogen mustard, a highly toxic agent with impressive activity in lymphoma and certain types of solid cancer, and methotrexate, developed by Sidney Farber in Boston, USA, and used from 1948 onwards for leukaemia, producing for the first time a worthwhile response rate, with durable remissions, in this dreaded childhood disorder.

Since that time, there has been an explosion of interest in all branches of cancer medicine, but perhaps most particularly in the use of anti-cancer chemotherapy agents which, even now, are finding new applications in cancer medicine. As little as twenty years ago, chemotherapy was still used only for a minority of cancers, whereas nowadays there are established or experimental chemotherapy protocols for virtually every type of cancer. Again, it must be remembered that there is an important distinction between novelty and progress, yet even the natural scepticism of the British medical establishment has begun to soften. As a form of cancer treatment, chemotherapy is very much here to stay, even for selected solid tumours with only partial responsiveness.

In Britain, it is customary for a single cancer specialist to be responsible for both the radiotherapy and chemotherapy administration, though many large treatment centres, including what many would regard as the best ones, are staffed both by specialists in radiotherapy (often nowadays termed 'clinical oncology') and also, separately, medical oncology; these latter specialists are concerned with chemotherapy administration and developmental aspects of chemotherapy. Elsewhere in the world, most notably the USA, medical oncologists actually outnumber radiotherapists (quite the reverse of the British situation) and for the most part, radiotherapists do not administer chemotherapy at all. It has to be said that, in most of the developed parts of Europe, the emphasis is more towards the American style of treating cancer, with separate specialists in clinical and medical oncology.

Although many non-specialists, such as general surgeons, general physicians and gynaecologists, do see and treat cancers, with varying degrees of competence but without further referral to a specialist, there is an increasing view (which I share) that patients with cancer really ought to have the opportunity of referral to a cancer specialist before firm treatment decisions are taken, even if surgical removal is the sole method of treatment required. This might also have the benefit of improving our rather dismal record of recruitment into clinical trials (see chapter 6). If the surgeon initially responsible for the diagnosis and surgical treatment does not suggest referral to a specialist, ask him or her. Everyone has the right to a second opinion, and who knows, it may lead to a change in policy or perhaps a more thorough assessment of the stage and other important features of the disease. I'm not suggesting that this is invariably the case – far from it – but some British specialists, particularly those who don't treat cancer actively themselves, do have a rather gloomy and negative view of the benefits of treatment, and some generalists might not even be aware of the latest advances in therapy, such as the rapidly increasing use of both radiation and chemotherapy as part of the treatment for certain categories of cancer of the large bowel. I'm all for the exercising of patient power, particularly when we have a newly commercialised health care system in the United Kingdom, with greater financial restraints on health authorities and hospitals than was previously the case, and, perhaps, an increasing disinclination to refer patients on for treatment that may be costly, but of uncertain benefit. My own view is that patients may have to be increasingly aggressive over the next decade or so, in order to get the advice and treatment which they have every right to expect.

Cancer surgery

Surgery remains an enormously important part of cancer treatment, though the role of surgery in some types of cancer has radically altered over the past twenty-five years. It is one of two main methods of establishing local control (the other being radiotherapy), and the surgeon has a unique contribution to cancer management in that he or she is potentially able to completely remove or debulk the primary site 'at a stroke'. If cancer was always a local disease, without the problem of distant metastatic spread, the cancer surgeon would doubtless reign supreme, as in the early part of this century, when heroic surgery was frequently undertaken. Surgery is still the most effective form of treatment for certain types of cancer, notably non-small cell lung cancer (see chapter 11), certain types of gynaecological cancer, e.g. early cancers of the cervix (chapter 14), many skin cancers, above all melanoma (chapter 18), most forms of soft tissue sarcoma (chapter 22) and gastrointestinal cancers (chapter 15). By and large, these are tumours in which no other method has yet proven to be superior to, or even the equal of, surgery, though in many cases – bone and soft tissue sarcomas are good examples – operations now are very much less radical than they used to be, since relatively conservative surgery, coupled with additional radiotherapy, chemotherapy or both, can provide as good a result in terms of survival, but with far superior functional results. Indeed, this general point holds true for much of cancer surgery today. In many areas, including genito-urinary and head and neck cancers (chapters 16 and 21), the use of early, post-operative radiotherapy has dramatically reduced the scope and extent of the surgical operation required. To give just one example, cancers of the larynx (voice apparatus) are now generally treated by radical radiotherapy (with or without chemotherapy) in an attempt to retain surgery as a secondary or 'salvage' approach, the intention, of course, being to retain the larynx and thereby the patient's normal speech function. Wherever possible, the surgeon and radio-therapist should work closely together to develop a recognition of the limits of each speciality in order to deliver the best possible service to the patient and to learn from both the successes and failures. Better, of course, to have a cured patient, even if the bladder or larynx has had to be removed, but better still if the patient is cured with the organs intact.

Perhaps the best example of all is in breast cancer, a disease which is unique in so many ways. Not only is it now the commonest of all female malignancies in the Western world, but most remarkably, policies for management have totally altered within the brief twenty-five year period from 1970. Mastectomy, so common up until that time, is now performed far more rarely, since the recognition that local tumour excision with breast preservation and early post-operative radiotherapy is at least the equal, in terms of overall survival figures, even to the most radical type of mastectomy. Secondly, we now have effective (or, to be accurate, 'partially effective') methods of reducing the likelihood of distant relapse through the use of either hormone or chemotherapy approaches. These points are discussed in more detail in chapter 12. Not all patients are suitable for the breast preserving approach, but with larger numbers of patients now seen with relatively small tumours detected by screening, patients who require mastectomy should become more and more unusual.

One of the paradoxes, however, is that a general surgeon is likely to be the first specialist that many patients with common cancers encounter, and we rely, of course, on the surgeon to take a proper biopsy and secure the diagnosis. Most surgeons are not only extremely competent and caring, but only too willing to co-operate with oncological colleagues who genuinely are cancer specialists. The traditional autocratic style of British surgeon is fast disappearing, but just occasionally, patients complain that they don't feel that the great cutter is a great communicator, and it may fall to others to carry the patient through an arduous series of investiga-tions and treatment. As hinted above, a further important role for the surgeon lies in the secondary or 'salvage' treatment of patients in whom every attempt has been made to produce a cure by non-surgical means, with full preservation of vital organs, but unfortunately has failed. Such patients aren't suitable for major surgical resection if they have already developed distant metastasis (secondary spread), but relapse at the primary site, a common problem for example in head and neck cancers, should very properly be treated in this way, with as much surgical reconstruction as is feasible. Indeed, reconstructive surgery, usually a joint endeavour between oncological and plastic surgeons, has an enormous contribution to make in cancer, either as part of the initial surgical approach, if major surgery is after all decided upon, or following salvage surgery of the type just mentioned. If salvage surgery is the only means of curing the patient, it should be very seriously considered, despite the drawbacks, since this may represent a genuine 'second chance'.

LASER SURGERY

Laser surgery is an exciting new departure which has become frequently used in the past ten years. Strictly speaking, it isn't surgery at all, at least not in the usual sense, but lasers can be used to remove blocks of tumour tissue, and are quite often used in accessible head and neck cancers, such as the tongue, as well as in removal of areas of early cervical cancer or pre-cancer. In recent years, very exciting advances have been made with laser treatment of lung and oesophageal (gullet) cancers, since conventional surgical treatment may be unsuitable, and the laser is capable of burning through completely blocked areas, then allowing local radiotherapy an opportunity for more long-term control. In cancer of the oesophagus, for example, patients quite often have such severe blockage that they may have lost more than ten per cent of their body weight and be unable to swallow any food at all. This dire situation can be rapidly reversed by laser application (easily repeatable if necessary), with re-establishment of the channel, relief of the blockage, and early treatment with radiotherapy. Although cure is extremely unlikely in such situations, excellent symptom response, sometimes with a durable remission, is usually achieved. At my own hospital we're also using lasers to deal with secondary liver deposits from colorectal cancer, by direct attack on these secondary metastases – in combination with chemotherapy.

The consequences of surgery for specific sites (for example the management of the patient after mastectomy and availability of prostheses and reconstructive services) are dealt with in specific chapters.

Radiotherapy and cancer

Although a much more youthful speciality than surgery, with a history stretching back only a hundred years, radiotherapy has become the pre-eminent form of cancer treatment and is now used for over fifty per cent of patients, this number steadily rising. Remarkably, the first attempt at using radiotherapy for skin and other cancers came within a few weeks of its discovery, and by 1924, the great British surgeon Sir Geoffrey Keynes had already started a systematic examination of its potential in breast cancer – happily he lived on to the age of ninety-four, quite long enough to see it established and also his prediction of the decline of mastectomy fulfilled. Improvements in radiotherapy equipment, technique and applications have led to an increasing role both in local treatment (in many cases, as outlined above, supplanting surgery or reducing the need for radical operations) and also in its use as a whole-body treatment, as part of bone marrow transplantation techniques for leukaemia and other malignant diseases (see chapter 20).

How does it work? X-rays and gamma rays lie at the most energetic end of the electro-magnetic spectrum, with a short wavelength and a high energy. Unlike all other energy waves, such as visible light, ultraviolet or radio waves, X-rays have sufficient energy to cause profound disruption of mammalian (including human) tissue cells through which they pass. Although this applies not only to tumour cells but also normal tissues, there is a real and exploitable difference between the limited capability of tumour cells to withstand the X-ray assault, and recover from it, and the much greater healing properties of normal tissues. Whether this difference is the result of an intrinsically greater radiation sensitivity by tumour cells or a superior power of recovery for normal cells remains somewhat in doubt. The net result, however, is that X-ray treatment of many cancers, when properly carried out with great attention to detail and dose requirements, can sterilise tumour tissue, often permanently, whilst producing a completely acceptable degree of local side-effects within the normal tissue surrounding it. A good example is in early cancer of the larynx (and fortunately the majority of cases of laryngeal cancer in the Western world fall into this category), a tumour in which radiation cure is achievable in over ninety per cent of cases, without any loss of function or serious injury to the voice. This figure is closely comparable with the degree of cure from surgery, but radiotherapy is much preferred, because of its greater degree of patient acceptability. Surgery is generally reserved (in the UK at least) for radiation failures.

The strategy of any radiotherapist is to try and achieve the best possible compromise between damaging the cancer cell and the normal surrounding host tissues. This is never easy, since a high dose of radiotherapy, often very close to the tolerance of normal organs, may have to be recommended by the radiotherapist in order to achieve a cure, particularly with the common solid tumours we treat every day (good examples include cancers of the cervix, bladder, prostate, breast and some types of lung cancer). The tragic case of radiation overdose described in Exeter in 1988, due to a simple failure of calibration of a new radiation source, demonstrated the serious, permanent damage that can occur when the radiation dose is as little as twenty-five per cent greater than it should be. I can't think of a single drug in common use in which the margin of safety is so slim. Likewise, the more recent and equally distressing discovery of systematic radiation underdosage occurring over a lengthy period at a hospital in Stoke-on-Trent confirmed that reduction of the total dose will also have serious consequences, this time due to failure of tumour control in a higher number of patients than one might reasonably expect. The radiotherapist constantly has to walk a very narrow tightrope between too low a dose, with failure to obtain the most out of what radiotherapy can offer (and a cure rate lower than it should be), and radiation overdose, with its unacceptable level of side-effects, some of which will result in long-term or even irreversible misery for the patient.

Over the past decade or so, tremendous advances in imaging techniques, notably with computer tomography (CT) and magnetic resonance imaging (MRI) have aided the radiotherapist in his or her task. For instance, before CT scanning was available, a patient with a malignant brain tumour who needed post-operative treatment generally required very wide field radiation therapy, in order to be sure of encompassing the tumour. Nowadays, with much improved tumour localisation, we can avoid the normal surrounding tissues more effectively, concentrating a higher dose more safely on the smaller volume we need to treat.

To complement improvements in tumour localisation, advances in both the quality and penetrating power of radiotherapy equipment have allowed us to deliver radiation to virtually any site in the body, with, for the most part, a uniform level of irradiation to the desired volume, and satisfactory fall-off in radiation dose outside the target volume. A much lower dose can be given to the surrounding sensitive tissues, in many cases with almost complete sparing of the skin – an important point, since it was this skin burning which so limited the radiation dose during the early part of the century. Individualised treatment plans have become commonplace, and techniques have now become much more sophisticated, with individually tailored shielding blocks to avoid treatment to sensitive areas such as the lung.

As well as treatment from outside the body ('teletherapy'), we can also deliver internal radiation therapy within the body, either by using a sealed source passed into a body orifice (or through the skin) and retained very close to the tumour site for the necessary period or, in some cases, by using a temporary or permanent radiation implant actually passed into the tumour itself. This is known as brachytherapy. Unsealed radiation sources, either swallowed or injected, are also available, and have very precise uses. In cancer of the thyroid, for example, we can exploit the fact that the thyroid gland is the only part of the body which will take up iodine (and therefore radioactive iodine as well) and deliberately give radioactive iodine by mouth, in the knowledge that it will immediately home in on the thyroid gland in the neck. Although the thyroid cancer cells never take up the iodine as well as the normal thyroid tissue, the first dose of the radioactive iodine will destroy the gland sufficiently effectively to allow a second dose, given some months later, to be taken up by the cancer cells, regardless of whether they are still contained within the gland area in the neck or have metastasised to other parts of the body, such as lung or bone. In this situation, radioactive iodine treatment can be highly effective even for patients with thyroid cancer which has spread well beyond the primary site. A true 'magic bullet' indeed! Other types of unsealed radioactive source are employed for malignant disorders of bone marrow, again exploiting the properties of certain radioactive agents to be taken up in the marrow, then destroying a portion of the adjacent bone marrow cells by direct radiation toxicity.

Radiation can be used with other types of cancer treatment as well, in combination with surgery, laser therapy, hormones or chemotherapy. Some cancers are routinely treated by a combination of external beam and implant therapy, the implant being used to boost the original tumour site to a high dose level, with the external beam treatment as a means of sterilising the microscopic secondary deposits which might be hidden in the local lymph node areas. As ever, the trick is to achieve maximum tumour cell destruction with minimal side-effects to normal tissues. In breast cancer (see chapter 12), radiation is given to the majority of patients who have undergone local excision and breast preservation, since the results of the local excision surgery alone are known to be less adequate in terms of local control of disease, to what could previously be achieved by mastectomy. Breast preservation is only possible because of the effectiveness of radiotherapy in sterilising small residual deposits of cancer within the breast, after the local excision operation has provided the major assault on the primary site. Fortunately, both these treatments are fully compatible with additional hormone therapy or chemotherapy.

Radiotherapy also has an important role in the treatment of most common solid cancers and in both Hodgkin's and non-Hodgkin lymphomas. Its role is more fully outlined in the specific site chapters. It also has an important role in the management of selected non-malignant tumours, such as benign pituitary gland or salivary tumours, though this important use of radiotherapy is not discussed further here.

There are some tumours in which radiotherapy was previously regarded as essential, but can now be safely avoided. Radiotherapy can be hazardous in childhood tumours because of growth retardation; most solid childhood cancers other than brain tumours are chemosensitive (i.e. responsive to chemotherapy), and radiotherapy is now used far less frequently in children, for example in those with non-Hodgkin lymphoma and Wilms' tumour (see chapter 24). However, the increased use of cranial (brain) irradiation, or, in some cases, treatment of both the brain and spinal cord has improved the overall cure rate for childhood brain tumours from about fifteen per cent to forty per cent. Furthermore, the use of growth hormone (now available in a fully biosynthetic form) and, if necessary, other hormone support, usually gives these children a near-normal final height and very good overall quality of life, in addition to cure of the tumour. In certain adult tumours, effective chemotherapy has also made radiotherapy less important, in some cases entirely redundant, as, for example, in the treatment of many testicular tumours and some types of lymphoma.

Radiotherapy is increasingly being used as a 'systemic' form of treatment, notably in combination with bone marrow transplantation. The idea here is that, for patients who have a poor outlook from certain types of malignant blood disorders such as leukaemia, multiple myeloma and lymphoma (particularly those in whom conventional methods have failed), it may be possible to perform a bone marrow transplant by using the patient's own bone marrow, if it can be sufficiently cleansed by chemotherapy or purged by other methods, removing it and treating the patient with high doses of total body irradiation and chemotherapy, in order to remove even the most resistant tumour cells. The marrow is then returned, repopulating the marrow space within the body and re-forming the essential bone marrow elements over the next few weeks. In other cases, it may be necessary to use donated bone marrow from a relative, if the donor and host tissues are sufficiently closely matched. This certainly ensures that the marrow will not be contaminated by residual tumour, but is very much more difficult in practice, because of the need to suppress immunity (since the graft is 'foreign' tissue) during the post-transplant period. Although it is the bone marrow transplant which is the 'glamorous' part of such treatments, it is, of course, the high doses of total body irradiation and chemotherapy which provide the real cure – the transplant simply provides the technological means of keeping the patient alive! More recently, it looks as though we might be able to do away with the transplant altogether, by using circulating blood cells stimulated by certain biological growth factors in order to bring out the powerful 'precursor' cells from the marrow into the bloodstream. With these techniques now widely available, it seems highly likely that the role and indications for total body irradiation and very high dose chemotherapy may extend rapidly over the next few years.

For patients with disease beyond the primary site, in whom cure is unrealistic, palliative radiotherapy is generally the most valuable of the treatments available, and is used in a wide variety of clinical settings, particularly for painful or unstable bone deposits. It can be used together with orthopaedic internal fixation, and these treatments are highly effective in rendering a patient both pain free and rapidly mobile. During the past decade, palliative treatments with radiotherapy have become much simpler, with a striking shift towards treatment with a smaller number of radiation fractions, but without any loss of effectiveness. In other clinical settings, where radical treatment is indicated, hyperfractionation techniques, i.e. treatment several times per day rather than the conventional one fraction per day approach, looks extremely promising and is being tested in clinical trial settings at present. Although it may have advantages for the treatment of well-localised tumours, for example in the head and neck, it certainly poses problems for any busy radiotherapy department, though a clear advantage, particularly to the patient, is the rapid completion of treatment in, say, two weeks instead of six.

Only a decade ago, many oncologists were predicting that improvements in chemotherapy and newer treatments were occurring so quickly that radiotherapy's great days were numbered; they argued that the systemic nature of most cancers meant that local treatments, however effective, would always remain inadequate and therefore become less important. Curiously, the reverse seems to have happened. Cure can never be achieved without control of the primary cancer. Obvious examples include cancers of the head and neck, prostate, bladder, cervix and large bowel – all areas in which the surgeon has previously dominated treatment. The management of breast cancer has undergone even more dramatic change. In my view, these developments will continue, and improvements in both radiological imaging and computer-assisted radiation targeting techniques will allow safer delivery of higher doses of radiation. This, in turn, should lead to improvements in local control.

Although we have clearly improved our ability to deliver effective radiotherapy without serious side-effects, we still have a long way to go. All too often, a radiation cure has its price in terms of both short and long-term toxicity. In the short term, acute effects, such a diarrhoea, skin discomfort and abdominal cramping from pelvic irradiation, should be relatively easy to deal with, particularly if short lived. It's the longer term side-effects which are so disturbing. For some patients (fortunately the minority), the price of a radiation cure for an otherwise lethal pelvic cancer (cervix, bladder and so on) can include long-term bowel damage, even leading to such severe radiation consequences that the affected part of the bowel has to be removed, and the patient provided with a colostomy. Sadly, all radiotherapists know that it is impossible to ensure that cure can always be achieved without the occasional case of severe damage of this kind – a consequence of biological variability within different patients. What this means is that some patients seem to have tissues which are more damaged than others by any given radiation dose. However, lowering the dose to a level which would never produce damage would reduce our radiation cure rate to an unacceptably low level as well.

Cancer chemotherapy and hormone therapy

In many ways, the development of hormone therapy and chemotherapy is the most exciting advance of all over the past forty years. Before the mid-1950s, patients with disseminated cancer, leukaemia or lymphoma invariably died of it. We now regularly expect to cure substantial groups of patients, including those with Hodgkin's disease, some of the non-Hodgkin lymphomas and leukaemias, many of the childhood cancers, and the majority of patients with testicular tumours. Even in more common conditions in which cure is still not possible, the advent of partly effective chemotherapy has meant an improvement in survival, often with lengthy remissions. This group includes ovarian cancer, myeloma, some of the non-curable lymphomas and some types of lung and breast cancer. Most exciting of all, perhaps, is the demonstration that in tumours like breast cancer, which are only moderately responsive to chemotherapy, its early use (as 'adjuvant' therapy), given directly after surgery, does clearly appear to improve the overall outlook with a statistically watertight improvement in survival documented as far out as ten years from diagnosis and initial treatment, even though the adjuvant chemotherapy had been completed many years before, and generally given for a total of only six months. This observation was the product of lengthy and painstaking international co-operation and speaks volumes for the enormous power of well-conducted clinical trials – a point discussed further in the next chapter. Clearly this has given the lead to workers in many other cancer areas, who naturally now wish to try and replicate this advantage by testing chemotherapy in other settings. Colorectal cancer, for example, is of considerable current interest because, like breast cancer, it is a tumour of relatively marginal chemosensitivity; yet early use of chemotherapy, when the tumour burden is at its minimum following surgical removal of the primary, seems again to be proving effective, though its track record so far is nowhere near as well documented as that of breast cancer.

CHEMOTHERAPY

Cancer treatment with effective cell-killing ('cytotoxic') therapy has much to contribute, yet the word 'chemotherapy' strikes dread into the hearts of many patients. It still seems to have a bad press, for two reasons: first, it was used far too indiscriminately in the early days, in the vain hope that it could cure every malignant ailment, however advanced. Secondly, it is still widely imagined that all patients receiving chemotherapy will inevitably suffer the most terrible consequences from side-effects.

We have moved on, I think, from the indiscriminate and largely valueless use of chemotherapy in situations where there could be no justification other than the physicians' desire to 'do something'. It has to be said that this was often fuelled by patients, though less so in Britain perhaps, than in other parts of the West, notably the USA, where the will to keep trying something new seems less tempered with an appreciation that, at some point, there has to be an end to active attempts at cure. With regard to chemotherapy side-effects, these too are much misunderstood. In the first place, only a small proportion of chemotherapy drugs cause really severe nausea and vomiting, and the good news is that, during the past five years or so, a new class of anti-nausea preparations, which seem to work by antagonising the trigger chemical causing nausea, have become widely available and have proven highly effective. Even powerful intravenous drugs, such as the platinum derivatives (see below) which can cause serious nausea and vomiting, are generally tamed by the new supportive anti-emetic agents. The second most feared side-effect, in my experience, is hair loss, which again is a feature of only a rather small proportion of chemotherapy drugs in common use. It is regrettable, of course – no one could pretend that it's a trivial matter to lose one's hair – but excellent wigs are available, hair loss (alopecia) is often only partial, and the best news of all is that the alopecia caused by cancer chemotherapy is invariably temporary; the hair always comes back, often wavier or curlier than before. Hair regrowth after cancer chemotherapy is one of the few absolute guarantees that the oncologist can give; indeed, I have even had the occasional male patient who was bald before chemotherapy and had significant hair regrowth afterwards!

The third major group of side-effects, bone marrow suppression ('myelosuppression') is a fairly consistent feature of cancer chemotherapy, but generally not to the point of danger. Again, advances in supportive drug therapy have greatly helped us, since it is not usually too difficult to tide the patient over a relatively temporary period of bone marrow failure. Anaemia can be relieved by blood transfusion if required; lowering of the white cell count (the anti-infection defence cells) can be countered by highly effective antibiotics and, if necessary, new biological growth factors; and a bleeding tendency from loss of the platelet cells of the blood is usually dealt with, if necessary, by platelet transfusions, which can be given until the danger period is passed.

Other types of chemotherapy agent have specific side-effects not shared by all of the drugs. For example, several of the drugs, notably the vincristine/vinblastine group (semi-natural drugs originally extracted from the periwinkle plant and known to act by inhibiting cell division), can cause a troublesome but reversible pins-and-needles/numbness syndrome by affecting the nerves in the hands and feet ('peripheral neuropathy'), while cisplatin, a chemically simple heavy-metal complex which has transformed many types of cancer (see below), can damage the kidney and cause deafness. We have learnt how to use these agents more safely, however – in the case of cisplatin, for example, by providing adequate hydration with intravenous fluids whenever it is used, and, if really necessary, by use of a cisplatin derivative drug (carboplatin) which has fewer of these side-effects. Pharmacologists, both in university settings, hospitals and the drug industry, have been extremely ingenious in recognising the limitations of current cancer chemotherapy and finding ways to overcome them.

A number of the anti-cancer drugs are sufficiently important to be worth describing in very brief outline here. For the most part, they fall into specific categories, with mechanisms of action which, in many cases, are reasonably well understood.

The inhibitory effect on tumour cell division of the periwinkle plant derivatives vincristine and vinblastine has already been mentioned. Some agents appear to act by inhibiting the DNA cleavage which precedes tumour cell division; they do this by tight binding of the DNA bases, thus preventing the chromosomal material within the tumour cell from being properly incorporated into the next generation of cells. Many of these drugs, such as cyclophosphamide, melphalan and busulphan, have been in common use for thirty years; many can be taken by mouth, and few have severe, long-term side-effects if taken in the correct dose. Some highly effective drugs are simple analogues or 'look-alikes' of biological base materials which would normally be incorporated into the DNA of an active tumour cell. These drugs, often termed 'antimetabolites' and frequently also available in tablet form, seem to work by being incorporated into the tumour cell base pairs which unite to form the tumour cell DNA; when cell division is attempted, the true nature of the cellular antagonist or 'look-alike' drug is revealed, and the DNA division is halted. The very simple agent 5-fluorouracil works in just this way, and there are many other similar examples.

Not all tumours respond to the same degree to the same chemical agents, and a number of principles are generally considered when the specialist decides that chemotherapy is required and has to select from the many drugs available. Increasingly, it is recognised that combination chemotherapy is superior to a single agent, presumably since this provides an opportunity for the tumour cells to be killed by a number of biochemical mechanisms working together. Preferably of course, drugs chosen for use in combination should be known to be active as a single agent for that particular tumour type; they should preferably have non-overlapping toxicities; they should be used intermittently, to allow normal tissue recovery; and ideally, each drug should be used in its optimal dose and schedule. Combination chemotherapy schedules (or 'protocols') generally employ agents from different categories of chemotherapy, in order to gain the maximum cell kill with a minimum of side-effects, and most chemotherapy specialists prefer to use well-established protocols or admit patients into clinical trials which will require proper documentation of responsiveness – one of the many advantages of trial work (see chapter 6).

As with radiotherapy, untoward consequences from chemotherapy can occur both in the short and long term. The acute side-effects already mentioned are generally brief in duration and manageable with standard methods of support – blood transfusion, antibiotics and so on. Long-term consequences are, on the whole, less severe than with radiotherapy, but can also be important and, again, may represent the price of cure. Most importantly, a number of these agents can cause infertility – not a problem for the majority of cancer patients, who are likely to be over forty years of age, but certainly a major issue in younger patients, including those with Hodgkin's disease and other lymphomas, whose prospect for cure may depend entirely on the effectiveness of chemotherapy if the disease is too widespread to be curable by local irradiation. Men, in particular, seem to be particularly affected in this respect, since the spermatic precursors (the cells from which mature sperms are derived) seem to be relatively easily damaged. Any young man faced with cancer chemotherapy for Hodgkin's disease or other conditions should therefore be warned about this and have the opportunity for sperm storage – an easy technological task, though some patients, particularly those with testicular tumours, have such a low sperm count that sperm banking proves impossible.

For women, the risk of infertility seems to be lower. With the increasing use of adjuvant chemotherapy for breast cancer, this has become one of the major uses of chemotherapy for women of child-bearing age, and all such patients should be warned that the chemotherapy might disturb the periods and could interrupt them altogether, without certainty of spontaneous recovery. In general, though, the younger the woman, the less likely she is to be rendered completely infertile, though I do always warn patients that they are likely to enter their menopause at an earlier age than might be otherwise expected, since a proportion of the ovarian tissue is likely to be permanently damaged by the chemotherapy. Sadly, it is not possible to store unfertilised eggs at present, in contrast to the easy storage of sperm. When it does occur, loss of fertility in female patients can have the most devastating consequences – this is discussed more fully in chapters 7 and 14.

Other long-term consequences of chemotherapy include permanent renal (kidney) damage, nowadays less of a problem since the main offending drug, cisplatin, is better understood and used more safely with adequate fluid hydration; and respiratory failure from cumulative dosage of the drug bleomycin, a widely used agent for testicular, head and neck and certain lung cancers. It is always tragic when successful cancer treatments are impaired by serious consequences of this kind, but it would be foolish to make recommendations regarding the specifics of drug administration, since each different tumour type may demand a different approach with several types of anti-cancer drug. Although chemotherapy is often at its most successful when used as part of a curative attempt, often given together with radical irradiation or surgery, it most certainly has benefits as palliative treatment as well, for example in patients with incurable breast, ovarian or small cell lung cancer. These points are discussed further in the specific chapters. As with so many aspects of cancer therapy, one of the most important treatment decisions concerns the issue of when to stop, when to say 'no more'. These decisions are at least as much cultural as medical, with a wide division of opinion between ourselves in the UK and our colleagues (and their patients, of course) in the USA. Perhaps at home in the UK we give in a little too gracefully, whereas in the USA the fault lies in the opposite direction.

When faced with the offer of chemotherapy for the first time, it is reasonable for the patient to ask, 'How much benefit and at what personal cost?' Specialists are there to answer questions just as much as to dish out the treatment, and most are only too happy to engage in an intelligent dialogue. In any event, even if they aren't keen, you, the patient, have a right to know. As so often in this book, my advice is: 'Don't just stand there, ask the question!'

HORMONE THERAPY

With hormone therapy, the situation is altogether different. Less widely used in cancer therapy, it is often seen as the 'gentler alternative' to chemotherapy. The truth is that its indications are much more limited, since only a small minority of tumours are hormone sensitive, including breast, prostate and uterus. As with chemotherapy, only a proportion of patients with these diseases respond, and it is generally impossible to determine in advance which these might be, with the exception of breast cancer, where we are able to use the reasonably reliable oestrogen receptor assay technique, which can be performed quite simply by staining the original biopsy material in the pathology department. Not all centres have this system in place, but frankly I don't feel that it is a crucial one, since some oestrogen receptor negative patients do respond to hormone therapy, and in general, the use of the most important hormone drug in breast cancer (tamoxifen) is so widespread (and the agent so low in toxicity) that detailed knowledge of the oestrogen receptor status of any individual patient may not be all that important. These points are discussed more fully in the specific chapters, but in general terms, the great advantage of hormone therapy is that it provides a systemic means of treatment, i.e. to the whole body, but without the side-effects of chemotherapy. Furthermore, hormone-induced responses are often remarkably durable, often more so than with chemotherapy. For example, in breast cancer, a highly hormone-sensitive patient with metastatic or secondary disease may enjoy years of good-quality life as a result of control of the secondary tumours by hormone manipulation, whereas chemotherapy in such circumstances tends to have a more short-lived effect. For this reason, even though response rates to hormone therapy in breast cancer are substantially lower than with chemotherapy, hormone therapy nonetheless tends to be preferred, for most patients relapsing for the first time. The anti-oestrogen tamoxifen, which is extremely active, is given by mouth to the majority of patients with breast cancer, has very few side-effects, and has been an established part of treatment for over a decade at least in post-menopausal patients. It has considerably improved survival and seems capable of reducing the risk of a contralateral primary, i.e. development of a new breast cancer on the other side. It is so active and relatively free of side-effects that it is now being used as a means of attempting prevention of breast cancer development in those regarded as being at high risk (usually by virtue of a very strong family history in an otherwise normal subject) – quite properly, within a randomised controlled trial setting.

chapter six

CLINICAL TRIALS ARE GOOD FOR YOU!

I freely admit that this is one of the areas of cancer medicine I feel most passionate about. Both in cancer and other medical specialities, the application of clinical trials has, in my view, been one of the greatest advances in scientific methodology and patient care since the Second World War. Too often in the past, medical treatments have been undertaken simply for traditional or historic reasons, but without the necessary scientific background that really proves their worth. How much better, for all concerned to discover that a new treatment really does work, proven by the most rigorous test of all, the prospective randomised controlled trial (about which more later). How many women, for example, were subjected to radical mastectomy between 1900 and 1970, on the assumption that it was an essential part of the cure of their breast cancer? We now know that, in the majority of cases, conservative surgical treatment, with full preservation of the breast and post-operative radiotherapy, produces an equally good result, at least from the point of view of control at the primary site. The extent of breast cancer surgery has no bearing whatsoever on the likely survival outcome. Yet the few brave souls who suggested this might be so were pilloried, almost burnt at the stake, for their heretical views. Traitors to the cause! But the truth is that the history of medical treatments is littered with ineffective remedies which were endorsed by the greatest medical men of the day, and therefore accepted as standard therapy. The same is true, of course, for cure-all alternative cancer remedies as practised by quack practitioners. One of the interesting features of cancer medicine is that, despite (or perhaps because of) its relatively short history, we are perhaps more dependent on the applications of truly scientific inquiry than any other branch of medicine – and a good thing too. It is surely simply a historical accident that both surgery and radiotherapy, for example, were introduced prior to chemotherapy. What we now need to do is to consider each of these separate techniques on their merits, without too much respect for the traditional approaches – unless, of course, they are supported by reliable scientific study, comparing the competing treatments.

Assessing the evidence

There are various levels of reliability in medical data and information.

ANECDOTE

First, at the lowest level, is the clinical anecdote – the individual patient story so beloved of tabloid newspapers, of the 'My grandfather smoked seventy cigarettes a day and lived to be ninety-two years old' variety. It is not that they are untrue, but simply that they can't be representative of any general truth or of more than passing interest. The absolutely unequivocal relationship between cigarette smoking and lung cancer is not diminished one jot by the narrative of the nonagenarian who smoked so enthusiastically, though it does remind us that, however strong the relationship, not all cigarette smokers develop cancer.

SMALL GROUP STUDIES

Next comes the study of a small group of patients treated in a similar way, and reported in the medical literature as 'clinical experience'. This, of course, is a major step forward from the clinical anecdote, since it implies a genuine spirit of inquiry on the part of the investigator, and an attempt to be consistent with respect to a novel treatment. The limitation, however, is that numbers are invariably very small, usually less than twenty patients, and most such studies are uncontrolled – i.e. have no comparison or 'comparator' group of similar patients who differ only in that the novel treatment was not available to them. The only possible treatment control, i.e. comparison with standard approaches, is by means of looking at a 'historical series'. Many trialists in cancer work are fond of this approach, since it does at least provide a pilot type of study for larger series of collaborative work, but even multi-centre studies involving hundreds of patients will, if limited to a single treatment group, suffer from the same shortcoming. Admittedly, the larger the number of patients (one real advantage of multi-centre studies, i.e. those coming from several institutes, is the more rapid development of a larger group of patients), the more statistical confidence we can have in the reliability of the result. A further advantage of this approach, making it popular in many parts of the world, is the ease with which such studies can be explained to the patient, who is simply asked whether he or she would agree to be considered for a novel form of treatment, since all other conventional approaches have failed in their particular case. Few patients have difficulty signing this type of consent form, and patient recruitment to such studies is often relatively rapid.

The difficulty, however, is that when one compares these patients to apparently similar ones treated, say, a few years beforehand, one immediately runs into a difficulty. It may well be that, over the same period that the new anti-cancer treatment was developed, there might also have been several advances in supportive care – antibiotic therapy, for example, or availability of blood product administration. There are a host of reasons why the two groups may not be strictly similar; indeed, the selection criteria for the patients in the study groups might have been subtly different in ways which even the investigator is barely aware of. If there does appear to be an improvement in disease recurrence, or, better still, survival, in favour of the new treatment, then it might wrongly be ascribed to the new cancer treatment, whereas, in fact, it could be simply the result of better supportive care, or even due to a slight but important difference between the groups of patients under study.

PROSPECTIVELY CONTROLLED RANDOMISED STUDIES

Far and away the most reliable means of detecting a genuine advance is the prospectively controlled randomised study. What does this ponderous term actually mean? The fundamental point is that the most important principle of all scientific experiments (as I learnt thirty years ago as an A-level science student) is that every detail of such an experiment should be held constant, with a single difference between the two study groups. This means that, if there is a genuine and reproducible difference in outcome, it must, as far as we can possibly tell, be due to that one variable. It may sound simple, but, of course, in terms of human biology and experimentation, the differences between any two individuals, their state of health and illness and their likely response to any treatment, are bound to be substantial. For this reason, individual patients are not sufficient, and we need to look at groups of patients in order to iron out any possible differences between them, as far as we are able. The greater the number of patients in each half of the study group, the more confident we can be that the biological differences are essentially erased, and that the groups of patients are therefore similar – apples and apples rather than apples and oranges. Essentially, this satisfies the first scientific criterion, that we have consistency throughout the system, but what about the introduction of the variable treatment? The essential point here is that prospectively randomised controlled trials deliberately allocate the new treatment *randomly* to half of the total group, whereas the other half is treated with the standard 'best buy' in terms of conventional, high-quality care. In well-designed randomised studies, all patients, whether in the 'new treatment' group or 'control' group, receive the best standard of care in any event, and half of them will be allocated the new treatment in addition. In this way, no possible bias can enter which might create two dissimilar groups.

Many criticisms have been made of this technique, but in my view, none of them erodes the central principle that this is by far the most powerful type of scientific study, capable of delivering a quality of data which is quite unparalleled by any other method. The first criticism is that this type of trial is somehow unethical, on the grounds that the specialist must surely have an idea what would constitute the best possible treatment for the patient, and therefore cannot reasonably enter his patients into a study where the treatment decision is made on the flip of a computerised coin, so to speak. The rebuttal, of course, is that, if the specialist really knew that a new treatment was better, it would indeed be unethical for him or her to enter such patients in the study; but it is because of the very uncertainty about the genuine benefit of a promising but unproven new treatment that the trial needed to be done in the first place. Secondly, what about the ethics of all this? Is it really right to make patients aware just how little we know and how uncertain the future might be? Or should we perhaps protect them and be cautious about informing them that a clinical trial is being performed because present techniques are unsatisfactory? I will return to this point later.

Criticisms of randomised trials

Critics of the prospectively randomised study complain that this type of trial is difficult to perform and often slow in patient recruitment. This can be true, particularly where the study is a multi-centre one, possibly funded by central agencies such as the Medical Research Council, who have very strict guidelines for the development of study protocols and the peer review process. It does indeed take time, and during that time, it is possible that a lesser type of 'one-arm' study, with historical comparison only, could have been completed and the results published. The difficulty is, however, that such studies rarely influence medical thinking to anything like the same degree as properly controlled clinical trials, simply because it is now widely recognised that the reliability of such studies is so limited.

Why should any patient agree to be enrolled into a clinical study of this kind, particularly if he or she is likely to have only a fifty per cent chance of receiving a promising new cancer agent, allocated at random? The first answer, in my view, is that any patient in a clinical trial, which has been proposed and carefully developed by experts in the field, reviewed and then refined before finalisation, is likely to be treated to the highest possible standards. Now that cancer treatments have become so complicated, this alone is an enormous advantage. All patients in the clinical study, whether allocated the new treatment or not, can be confident that their care will be of the highest quality. Secondly, new treatments have a habit of being promising in the early stages, but less impressive when tried out in large numbers of patients later on. The development of cancer care has mostly been one of painstaking, slow research, chipping away at difficult problems rather than dramatically advancing with a sudden breakthrough. Such events are extremely unusual. The promising new agent may turn out to be more detrimental, by virtue of troublesome, unexpected side-effects, than beneficial. For every successful clinical trial, there is another which produces a negative result, sometimes even showing benefit for the 'control' rather than the 'new treatment' group.

One further real advantage for patients participating in these studies is that, although they may or may not receive a new treatment which turns out to be active and worthwhile, they are making a real contribution to medical care, of possible benefit to those who, like them, will be suffering in later years from an illness that could, at present, be incurable. Many patients are cheered and pleased by this knowledge; indeed, the altruistic element of co-operation is quite common in my experience. Many women with breast cancer, for example, feel a sense of comradeship with fellow sufferers, and are also aware that, as the disease is to some extent familial, their own daughters and granddaughters might be affected and could benefit from their own participation in a clinical trial.

RANDOMISATION

The most difficult ethical problems in randomised studies concern the very fact of randomisation, and the question of informed consent. Randomisation itself must seem a very blunt instrument, given the way in which the public holds dear the advice of the medical profession, advice which is generally felt to be the result of lengthy study and endless hours walking the wards to gain clinical experience. Whilst this may be flattering, it is as well to remember that, in a disease as frequently fatal as cancer, what we don't know is regrettably much more than what we do. Even where we may have a highly effective treatment – tamoxifen for breast cancer, for example – we still don't know how long patients should receive it for, and no amount of 'clinical experience' can substitute for the asking of a simple scientific question. At present the Cancer Research Campaign in the UK is quite properly addressing this, allocating patients to two years or five years of treatment with this agent, in a randomised controlled trial setting, to see which is preferable. It may be that five years is better than two, and this certainly seems to be the intuitive expectation of many patients and doctors, but equally it could be the case that the two years' exposure, which we already know (from previous randomised trials, of course!) to be superior to no tamoxifen at all, is as good as one can get. The additional three-year treatment may result more in extra side-effects than in further benefit. We just don't know. Despite this, many specialists, without any evidence at all, recommend tamoxifen for their breast-cancer patients 'for life' on the grounds that what is good for you over a two-year period must be good for you long term. Who knows? We need to do the studies to find out, and it is worth bearing in mind that very few, if any, treatments in medicine come free, so to speak; even the most innocuous of drugs generally turn out to have at least some side-effects, so it's a question of balancing these against the advantages of lengthier treatment.

Some have argued that the randomisation step can be substituted by some other form of dividing the two groups, for example the allocation of patients either to the control or treatment arm in a strict alternating sequence, as they walk through the clinic door, so to speak. This seems to me to highlight the very real dangers inherent in any type of trial which is not truly randomised. Consider, for example, the use of a promising new chemotherapy type of agent or new type of radiotherapy technique. The enthusiastic designer of the study will be armed with the knowledge that patient number one who walks in will be allocated the new experimental treatment (which of course, in his heart of hearts, the doctor might think to be better than the old). In walks patient number one, a fit, youngish individual with an appropriate kind of tumour; he is promptly entered into the study. In walks patient number two, less fit looking, perhaps, but quite acceptable as a control patient. Patient number three is less fit still, and the investigator knows in advance that he will receive the new treatment, if entered into the study at all! 'I don't think he's quite suitable, on the grounds of general state of health,' he murmurs to himself as he shakes his head and waits for the next patient, to see whether he might be fit enough to be considered. In this way, it is easy to imagine how bias can enter the system, producing a very much fitter group of patients for the new treatment than for the control arm of the study. Three years later, a real difference in survival has emerged, wrongly attributed to the new treatment, and the successful trialist receives many plaudits and invitations to speak all round the world. Poorly controlled clinical trials can be extremely damaging.

INFORMED CONSENT

The other knotty problem, so far not solved to anyone's satisfaction, is the issue of informed consent. As Professor Souhami and I recently pointed out in an article in the British Medical Journal:

> *'One of the most important ethical and practical difficulties in randomised clinical trials concerns the nature of informed consent. Every patient has the right to be treated in the best possible way for his or her condition and to be as well informed as he or she wishes about the possible approaches available. On the other hand, there is the urgent need to validate new treatments. The conflict that may arise between these positions has resulted in many cancer physicians feeling (and expressing) considerable anxiety about the constraining effects of the informed consent procedure as an essential prelude to a patient's participation in clinical trials, particularly randomised clinical trials.*
>
> *The issue of informed consent has thus become a major barrier to the*

successful conduct of randomised clinical trials with cancer. The many practical difficulties have led to low levels of recruitment, especially where there is a substantial difference between the treatment policies being compared. In our judgement, the medical profession has been unnecessarily defensive and, by and large, has failed to point out that the ethical positions which have been generally accepted are themselves contradictory and impractical. In our view, attempts to gain the "informed" participation of patients in randomised clinical trials are already doing harm in many individual cases.' ≥●

'Fully informed consent' means different things to different investigators (and patients, of course) but essentially it implies a full discussion of the various treatment alternatives with every patient who is being asked to participate in the clinical study, regardless of whether they might be allocated the new treatment or control (traditional treatment). This leads, for example, to a lengthy discussion with all patients of the pros and cons of the new treatment, even though only fifty per cent of the group will receive it. As Souhami and I pointed out in our paper,

≥● *'It is neither faintheartedness nor a disinclination to be questioned that discourages the clinician; rather, it is the overwhelming difficulty of describing the details of a potentially valuable (but as yet unproved) new remedy, gaining the patient's assent, and later having to inform her that she has been randomised to receive radiotherapy alone (rather than, say, radiotherapy plus chemotherapy, which is a promising but not fully established method of treatment for carcinoma of the cervix). However carefully the pros and cons of chemotherapy may have been explained, the result of the randomisation often leads the doctor towards a rather shabby display of back-pedalling, in which the possible advantages of the chemotherapy are "talked down" and perhaps the side-effects "talked up". The patient may become extremely distressed, which is not only counterproductive (with refusal to participate) but also alarming to the doctor and by no means easily resolved. It does not take many such consultations to change a well-intentioned and committed trialist into a disgruntled clinician who no longer feels that the game is worth the candle. It can be extremely difficult to sustain the doctor-patient relationship through such a harrowing discussion, and particularly unfortunate for patients such as those in the example above whose treatment by radiotherapy (that is, the control group) would be regarded as entirely conventional and proper. Both the support and reassurance of the doctor, and the patient's trust and confidence in the medical advice, may have been irretrievably lost. Too frank an explanation, with patient overload from too much information, can have most serious consequences.'* ❧

In other words, the insistence on fully informed consent is both counterproductive in terms of recruitment to important clinical studies, but also unnecessarily cruel in human terms, since it's as if the carrot of a potentially valuable new treatment has been dangled in front of the patient, then snatched away after they have reached out for it by agreeing to participate in the study in the first place! This seems to me ethically dubious, to say the least, and despite being a very committed clinical trialist, I don't find it easy to pursue this approach. What might, I think, be more realistic would be an acceptance that not all patients wish to know every last detail; indeed, not all are necessarily capable of grasping every nuance of what is said to them. Why shouldn't the doctor be the best judge of just how much information to impart? After all, this is precisely what he or she does in normal clinical practice. Providing information to patients is often a matter of pacing the discussion over weeks or even months. Of course, there will be patients who wish for full disclosure of the details of the study, including any randomisation steps in the decision-making process, and I am more than happy to discuss these fully. But equally there are those who are happy to place their trust in the doctor in the traditional way, and I'm not sure that it is ethically permissible to thrust unwelcome facts at them. In between, of course, there are all shades of intelligence, concern and trustfulness, and doctors undertaking clinical trial work should be sensitive to the differing needs to their patients. After all, most clinicians recognise that the anxious patient sitting opposite them in the consulting room requires, above all, reassurance and a clear explanation of what needs to be done to provide a cure. An increasing degree of frankness on the part of the doctor, for the most part laudable and constructive, may cause considerable anxiety in patients who would prefer to be directed rather than to participate as an equal partner. It might surprise many to know that this group of patients may include highly sophisticated professionals, for instance the late Dr Franz Ingelfinger, for many years the editor of the *New England Journal of Medicine* (probably one of the most prestigious medical journals), shortly before his death from cancer. Having been diagnosed as suffering from a potentially terminal illness, he wrote:

❧ *'I received from physician friends throughout the country a barrage of well-intentioned but contradictory advice . . . as a result, not only I but my wife, my son and daughter-in-law (all doctors) and other family members became increasingly confused and emotionally distraught. Finally, when the pangs of indecision had become nearly intolerable, one wise physician friend said, "What you need is a doctor." He was telling me to forget the information I already had . . . and to seek instead a person* who would tell me what to do, who would in a paternalistic manner assume responsibility for my care. *When this excellent advice was followed, my family and I sensed immediate and immense relief. The incapacity of enervating worry was dispelled, and I could return to my usual anxieties, such as deciding on the fate of manuscripts.'* ✌

Clinical trials really are good for you! They ensure that you are treated to the highest possible standards of care, they allow you to make a genuine contribution which may benefit not only yourself, but also many others, and they ensure that the results of your treatment will be carefully documented and analysed. Regrettably this is not by any means the rule in non-trial situations. Most clinical trials are held together by an enthusiastic working party and a trial co-ordinator who travels around the country to the various centres ensuring that the data is kept absolutely up to date and ready for proper statistical analysis. The importance of controlled clinical trials in cancer cannot be over-emphasised, and they have certainly proven immensely influential, increasingly taken up by the media and rapidly disseminated, provided the quality of data is strong enough. All of us in the health service have become accustomed to the concept of auditing our treatment outcomes and, in my view, the controlled clinical trial is the best possible form of medical audit!

I believe that patients with cancer should always ask their specialist whether there are any clinical trials currently taking place in his or her department (or nationally, to which he or she might be a contributing clinician) so that they can decide whether or not they wish to participate. If 'patient power' means anything at all, it surely means providing an opportunity for patients to ask questions, to be pro-active, to recognise that it is their life, not the clinician's, which is at stake, and to seek the best possible standard of care. As for cancer clinicians, I feel that they should remember the title of one the keynote addresses at the 1995 Harvard Medical School annual celebrations: 'Research is an obligation, not an option'.

7

SUPPORTIVE CARE AND THE QUALITY OF LIFE

M any of the standard cancer treatments currently available are undeniably tough on the patient. Whether or not he was the first to point it out, Shakespeare was surely right when he noted, 'Desperate diseases by desperate means are cur'd/Or not at all,' and it is true, as pointed out in previous chapters that both radiotherapy and chemotherapy may have to be given intensively, with the possibility of unwelcome side-effects, to be effective. Perhaps, after all, Shakespeare missed his true vocation: he was a cancer physician *manqué*.

Since we are stuck with beneficial treatments which cause side-effects in quite a high proportion of our patients, we have had to find methods of alleviating these problems as far as possible. During treatment, patients are likely to require a whole variety of supportive remedies to get them through the treatment in the safest possible way. In addition of course, their psychological state of mind is bound to be disturbed, to say the least, and we can only hope that family, friends and professional counsellors can provide at least some of the reassurance, love and support needed. Many find it comforting to know that they are not alone in their anguish and fears, and many patients find mutual self-help support groups, run by those who have been through the same thing themselves, more valuable than even the most devoted attentions of their closest partners and family.

Post-treatment consequences

Following surgical operations for cancer, the recovery period is usually fairly rapid, depending of course on the site, extent and scope of the surgery. Many patients are out of hospital within a week or so following standard procedures such as mastectomy, hysterectomy or exploratory abdominal operations. Other operations inevitably take longer – removal of a lung (pneumonectomy) or a bowel resection (hemicolectomy), for instance. Major and complicated operations, particularly those in the head and neck region which require surgical reconstruction, are inevitably more taxing and generally require a longer period both in hospital and for recovery. Complex procedures are generally best undertaken at special centres where the appropriate teams of surgeons, working in co-operation, are available – and well used to working with each other.

Always ask your surgeon about the likely consequences of an operation and how long it will take for recovery. It might also be a good opportunity to let the surgeon know that whatever the outcome, you would like to hear the results of the operation and to know about what the pathologist found when he or she examined the specimen. You may not wish to do this; of course, but many patients feel inhibited from asking these questions, since they feel 'it's not their place' even though they would like to have the information. This simply won't do! You have to be bolder than that if you want to participate in your care and be kept well informed. You may not wish to, of course, and I'm not saying you *have* to, but there is no need to feel that information about your own body, your own state of health, is somehow not your business.

When it comes to more specific cancer treatments, such as radiation and chemotherapy, patients are generally warned in advance that they might suffer certain consequences. One real difficulty in this area concerns the question of just how far the specialist should go in warning patients of potential undesirable consequences. If, for example, a radiation side-effect is virtually universal, such as hair loss following irradiation for a brain tumour, it would be wholly wrong and unfair to fail to warn the patient, though advising different individuals as to how long it might take before re-growth occurs is always a problem, since it can be highly variable dependent both on dose, age of the patient and other factors. If, on the other hand, a complication is extremely unusual, but very occasionally occurs, should one frighten every patient by pointing out that it could happen? A good example of this, much discussed in the media recently, concerns the radiation damage, particularly the arm weakness, that can occur as a result of irradiation of nervous tissue during radiotherapy treatment for breast cancer. A very small proportion of the total number of treated women – probably of the order of less than one in a thousand across the country – has developed profound weakness of the arm, in a minority of cases to the point of incapacity or even amputation to provide relief. Should all patients be warned about this? Would it do more good than harm? Might they unwisely forgo a critically important part of their treatment because of an unreasonable fear? These are not easy questions, particularly since many radiotherapists will never have seen a single case in their own personal practice, over many years' work in the field.

Perhaps the patient should decide, when meeting the radiotherapist for the first time, just how much he or she wishes to know about the potential dangers, as well as the possible benefits, of the treatment being proposed. Obviously no radiotherapist would treat a patient unless the benefits are likely to outweigh the disadvantages, but the patient may well need reassurance on this point and may, at the end of the day, take a different view. It is extremely unfortunate to cure a patient of cancer and yet face their anger and dismay if a serious radiation side-effect has developed, which they may feel they were not adequately warned about.

Serious radiation damage is fortunately rare, though the need to keep dosage high for best tumour effect does, of course, mean that side-effects of moderate severity are often encountered. In irradiating tumours of the head and neck, for example, large volumes of the lining of the mouth and/or throat may have to be treated, with irritation, soreness and dryness of these surfaces commonly occurring as an acute reaction. The pain may be so intense that patients cannot easily swallow, requiring liquid diets, nutritional support, and even nasogastric tube feeding or a specially positioned stomach tube (gastrostomy). These methods of support can make all the difference to a patient who would otherwise not be able to withstand such treatment without severe weight loss. In my experience, these methods of support are often essential since, for a patient with locally advanced cancer in the head and neck region, there is still a chance of cure, even without surgery, provided that the radiation (and, in some instances, chemotherapy) is given in a sufficiently intensive dose. As so often, it is the supportive care which makes possible the full delivery of the scheduled anti-cancer treatment.

Radiation therapy for lung cancer may also cause difficulties with swallowing, because of the direct radiation effect on the oesophagus (gullet). It is usually possible to keep the patient going during treatment, using antacid and other soothing medicines such as mucaine, which lines the oesophagus and gives a soothing local anaesthetic effect. Most radiotherapy departments run a strict policy of assessing each patient (by a doctor) at least once per week, regularly throughout treatment – this is your opportunity to let the specialist know whether these kinds of symptoms are developing, so that he or she can deal with them before they become too severe.

In the abdomen, the limited radiation tolerance of many of the organs, such as liver, small bowel, kidney and so on, has led to a particularly cautious use of radiotherapy. The abdomen essentially remains the province of the surgeon when it comes to primary treatment, though many tumours metastasise to various organs within this body cavity, and secondary treatments, generally with some form of chemotherapy administration, are commonly attempted. In the pelvis, radiation has an extremely important role both in gynaecological tumours (particularly cervix and uterus) and for genito-urinary sites, such as bladder and prostate. Because of the proximity and radiation tolerance of the lower bowel (rectum) and other structures close by, this is an exceptionally difficult site in which to achieve in every case the ideal compromise between under- and overdosage. The patient's life is all too often genuinely at stake, since the treatment (generally by radiotherapy, but sometimes with a combination of radiation and chemotherapy) represents the only possible chance of cure since many of these patients unfortunately have an inoperable disease.

On the other hand, it is tragic indeed to produce severe side-effects where the patients might have been curable without them, though in the individual case it can, admittedly, be virtually impossible to determine whether this happy outcome might have been possible. Rectal bleeding, continued discharge, pelvic pain, diarrhoea and fistula formation are all possible consequences, though not always due simply to the treatment. Fistula formation (a fistula is an abnormal opening between two adjacent organs, such as the bowel and bladder) may result from radiation damage, but also occurs if there is tumour regrowth. In such cases, it may be necessary to divert the bowel and provide a long-term colostomy, in order to prevent contamination of the bladder area by faecal material. In the case of a fistula between the bladder and vagina, also occasionally a consequence of high-dose radiation to the pelvis, the patient will leak urine from the vagina, and a ureteric diversion (i.e. surgical removal of the ureters from the bladder, then implanting them onto the abdominal wall, to allow the urine to escape into an ileostomy bag) will need to be performed so that the patient can be dry again. This is dealt with in more detail in chapter 16.

These undesirable consequences of radiation do occur from time to time, even in the best hands – unless, of course, the therapist is prepared to lower the radiation dose and accept more treatment failures as the price of never causing this type of damage.

Complications of chemotherapy

Although chemotherapy has traditionally had a bad press from the point of view of severity of side-effects, enormous improvements have been made over the past ten years in the alleviation of such symptoms. In particular, the treatment of chemotherapy-induced emesis (nausea and vomiting) and of the bone marrow consequences (leading to dangerous reduction of the circulating blood elements) is now much more effective.

Since most forms of chemotherapy act to some extent as cell poisons, it is perhaps not surprising that nausea and vomiting are such frequent symptoms. In truth, however, the reason for chemotherapy-induced emesis is poorly understood, though there appears to be a centrally located chemotherapy trigger zone mediated by neurochemical transmitters in the brain (i.e. the production of chemically active substances, which are potent causes of vomiting when released and recognised within a specific part of the brain). Recognition of this mechanism, with the appropriate development of antagonists to the neurochemical transmitter substances, has been highly successful in producing a new class of agents which are far more potent as anti-emetics than those previously available. Most chemotherapy agents are capable of causing this distressing side-effect, with three particular drugs, doxorubicin (Adriamycin), cisplatin and nitrogen mustard (mustine) as the worst offenders. Most of the drugs which can be given by mouth, such as cyclophosphamide, busulphan, melphalan and methotrexate, are less likely to cause severe nausea.

With the available anti-nausea drugs – generally a combination of potent steroid agents such as dexamethasone and specific anti-nauseants such as metoclopramide (Maxolon), prochlorperazine (Stemetil) and domperidone – most patients treated with moderately nauseating chemotherapy are well enough supported to cope pretty well, and even to get back to work within a day or two of the chemotherapy administration.

With the more powerful group, the newer agents, which are antagonists of the neuro-transmitter substance serotonin (also known as 5-hydroxy-tryptamine or 5HT) are extremely effective, though still rather expensive and only recently introduced. The two most commonly used agents in this category are ondansetron (Zofran) and granisetron (Kytril). They have certainly transformed many patients' acceptance of powerful but highly nauseating drugs such as cisplatin. Bone marrow suppression is, if anything, a more serious problem, less upsetting for the patient perhaps, but potentially far more dangerous. Most of the chemotherapy drugs do cause some degree of temporary bone marrow failure (myelosuppression), fortunately short lived in the majority of cases. However, just as radiation oncologists are rightly obsessed by delivering the proper dose for the best possible effect, specialists in cancer chemotherapy are also extremely concerned that high doses should be given wherever possible, since this is likely to lead to a much-improved response. The traditional barrier to such high-dose treatment has been the inability of the bone marrow to cope with it, leading to dangerous periods of neutropenia (suppression of the white cells that are essential for defence against infection) and thrombocytopenia (reduction in the platelet count, leading to bruising and bleeding). Anaemia does, of course, also occur, but is generally easily reversible by blood transfusion.

Traditionally, careful attention to early treatment of the infectious episodes during neutropenia and/or early platelet transfusion has been the major means of combating myelosuppression, and the development of potent new generations of antibiotic has been extremely valuable. In patients with fragile bone marrow reserve, such as those with acute leukaemia, it is particularly important to treat with an antibiotic, generally by intravenous administration, if the patient is neutropenic and develops a fever, even before the infectious cause of that fever has been established, since there is simply no time to lose. In patients with solid tumours, whose bone marrow reserve is normal, one can usually be a little more relaxed, assuming, of course, that conventional doses of anti-cancer chemotherapy have been given and that early bone marrow recovery can confidently be predicted.

Our ability to deliver higher doses with safety has been considerably advanced by the development of biological substances, generally known as cytokines, which are bone marrow stimulators of various types. These agents enhance our own bodily defences, assisting the natural substances which would normally be responsible for bone marrow recovery after a drug-induced temporary failure of the type produced by cytotoxic ('cell-killing') chemotherapy. Most of these 'biological response modifiers' work on the white cell series and are generically known as CSFs (colony stimulating factors). We currently have at least two important agents available, one of which stimulates granulocytes (G-CSF) – granulocytes being the most potent white cell defence against bacterial infection – and the other capable of stimulating both granulocytes and a second white cell sub-population, the macrophage series (GM-CSF). An increasing number of biological factors have now been shown to have an influence on haemopoietic (blood and marrow) cell growth and differentiation. Both the CSF series, and also other drugs known as interleukins, have an important effect on red and white cell development in the bone marrow and elsewhere, and many are currently undergoing clinical study. There also appear to be inhibitory substances (including some of the inter-leukins) which might have a role in protecting these haemopoietic progenitor cells, or possibly even cells of the gastro-intestinal epithelium (the lining of the intestine) at the time of chemotherapy. Several controlled clinical studies have now shown a benefit following the use of G-CSF during intensive chemotherapy, involving intensive che-motherapy for small cell lung cancer and non-Hodgkin lymphoma. These randomised studies have shown that the use of G-CSF is generally associated with reducing the incidence or duration of neutropenic fever, but no studies have yet shown an overall survival advantage. Attempts to improve the early recovery of platelets have been less successful, though fortunately, platelet transfusions are freely available and are generally capable of tiding patients over brief periods (i.e. less than a month) of severe thrombocytopenia.

It is difficult to overestimate the value of high-quality supportive care for patients undergoing cancer treatment. Careful attention to nutrition, psychological support, appropriate anti-emetic therapy and early treat-ment of fever, particularly during periods of chemotherapy-induced neutropenia, have all been highly contributory in producing the best possible results. However, where conventional cancer chemotherapy is unlikely to produce a cure, more powerful methods of treatment have to be found. Chief among these at present is the use of bone marrow transplantation, originally introduced for leukaemia, but now much more widely used, in order to increase dose intensity with an acceptable margin of safety for the patient. The theory is essentially twofold. First, if patients with leukaemia or similar disorders were to undergo very intensive chemotherapy (sometimes with whole body irradiation as well) in order to deliberately ablate (suppress to the point of zero function) their bone marrow, then transplantation of matched mar-row, generally from a sibling, might safely be able to repopulate the recipient's marrow with the leukaemia completely destroyed by the highly intensive chemo-radiotherapy. Secondly, an alternative approach both for leukaemia, lymphoma and some of the more refractory solid tumours might be to remove part of the patient's own bone marrow (hopefully uncontaminated with malignant cells, as would be the case with most solid cancers, or if previously involved, cleared of tumour cells as far as possible by conventional chemotherapy), then give very high-dose chemotherapy (again, possibly with total body irradiation as well), then finally return the patient's own marrow, once again. The first technique is known as allogeneic bone marrow transplantation, and the second as autologous transplantation. The former is a much more dangerous, though often curative, procedure, whereas the latter, with no risk of transplantation mis-match (after all, it is the patient's own marrow that is removed and then returned) potentially has very wide applications in cancer work. It could prove to be the most logical means by which much more intensive chemotherapy might safely be given to partly responsive solid tumours. Indeed, there is already some evidence that in certain tumours, such as Hodgkin's disease, the non-Hodgkin lymphomas and refractory testicular tumours, such techniques have produced cures where the patient would otherwise have died.

The use of autologous bone marrow transplantation has certainly allowed us all to become much bolder in our use of higher chemotherapy dosage, thus widening the potential of successful treatment for a far larger patient group. Even more exciting, perhaps, is the development over the past two or three years of peripheral blood stem cell transplantation (PBSC), which is beginning to replace autologous bone marrow transplantation entirely. In this technique, the patient's bone marrow is stimulated either by chemotherapy or CSF-type cytokines, with the effect of stimulating early marrow precursor cells into the circulating or peripheral blood. These can then be collected, concentrated and used as support for high-dose chemotherapy. The technique can be repeated and much higher doses of chemotherapy safely given. Clearly, this may be an effective way forward in breast, lung and other common solid cancers, but we will have to wait for the results of randomised studies addressing this issue. The availability of new technology is rapidly outstripping our ability to test them all thoroughly – only a few years ago, autologous bone marrow transplantation was very much the vogue, whereas it is now rapidly being discarded in favour of PBSC collection.

Quality of life issues in cancer

No one would dispute the fact that, to achieve a cure from cancer, most patients would be prepared to put up with almost any degree of treatment-related side-effects, provided they came through in the end. Whilst it is certainly justifiable to put patients through a very tough time if there is simply no alternative to achieve a cure, what about patients for whom cure is only a remote possibility? How do we help them, yet make sure that in our enthusiasm to do what we can, we don't do more harm than good?

Oncologists have long been aware of this dilemma; indeed, some of the earliest studies in Hodgkin's disease, dating from the 1960s, recognised the extremely nauseating effects of the relatively primitive (but sometimes effective) chemotherapy, and attempted to substitute effective, but less nauseating, drugs for the worst offenders. This has led to newer and more acceptable regimens for Hodgkin's disease which are substantially still in use today. Although the newer treatment is no better in terms of effectiveness, it is certainly far less emetogenic (nauseating) and therefore much more acceptable to patients. More recently, those interested in the quality-of-life area have attempted to define methods of measuring this elusive component of our daily lives (everyone knows what it means but few can put it exactly into words!). Generally, these assessment techniques depend on patient questionnaires, but there are also methods by which patients enter a mark on a simple linear analogue scale ('How well do you feel today, on an arbitrary scale of 1 to 10?'). This technique can be expanded to cover many specific questions concerning mood, physical comfort, freedom from specific complaints, such as nausea, breathlessness, constipation and so on, and many other areas.

The whole topic is brilliantly dealt with in Dr Lesley Fallowfield's book *The Quality of Life*, which both addresses the general issues of the quality of life and also takes doctors to task for quite frequently disregarding it. It is certainly important to recognise at all times whether one's enthusiastic use of dangerous and discomforting drugs is always justified, particularly in diseases like extensive small cell lung cancer (see chapter 11) where cure is only a remote possibility. It is far more important to recognise that the patient's quality of life, given that the total time is likely to be limited, is of much greater importance perhaps than a few extra weeks. Needless to say, patients do vary considerably in their views on this matter, and some prefer every attempt to be made regardless of personal cost, particularly if they wish to remain alive, as so often seems the case, for a particular event, such as the birth of a grandchild, a daughter's wedding and so on. Many patients are quite frank about these matters, and rightly expect a corresponding degree of candour on the part of the physician treating them. Most patients much prefer honesty, even if the news is disappointing, to evasiveness or an elaborate discussion cloaked with half truths. It is all to the good that, during the past decade, there has been increasing attention to the quality of life in patients undergoing cancer treatment. For many patients, quality of life is highly dependent on their physical condition, and every attempt should be made to reduce the negative and highly debilitating side-effects of cancer. One European oncologist with a particular interest in this area has recently written:

> *'Conceptually, quality of life has to do with the sense of satisfaction and well-being that an individual feels about his or her life, encompassing qualities such as the degree to which an individual succeeds in accomplishing his desires, and the extent to which a person's hopes and ambitions are matched and fulfilled by experience.'* [1]

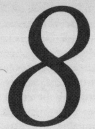

8

NEWER APPROACHES: BEWARE THE BREAKTHROUGH

Probably more than in any other medical speciality, oncological research attracts a remarkable degree of central and industrial funding, public interest and media exposure. Many clinicians groan with despair at yet another 'New Breakthrough in Cancer' headline since the following day's clinic is likely to be considerably slowed down by patients clutching the newspaper cutting! A difficult task is made still more challenging by having to disappoint them, but the truth is that most cancer breakthroughs are reported far too early, generally at the stage when the researchers have cautiously announced the preliminary findings. Even the broadsheet newspapers are far from immune from trumpeting apparent successes far too soon.

The role-call of treatments which have been subjected to this dizzy elevation is a lengthy one; a select list might include 'All Leukaemia to Be Cured by Drug Therapy before 1990', 'Bone Marrow Transplantation the Answer for Solid Tumours as well [as leukaemia]', 'Chemo-hormone Treatment Halves Death Rate in Breast Cancer', 'Magic Bullet Radiation Cures Ovarian Cancer', 'Interferon Therapy Set to Decimate Cancer Deaths' and so on.

The frustrating part is that these reports often contain a germ of truth. It's not much more than twenty years ago, for example, that bone marrow transplantation came into increasing use as a serious option for patients with refractory leukaemia who might otherwise have expected only a few months' survival. Prior to that, it had been regarded as a crack-pot idea, yet another example of an ill-judged medical technology being applied in an impossible situation, mostly for the aggrandisement of the haematologist. Now thousands of patients in the UK and elsewhere owe their lives to this technique, and high-dose chemotherapy, sometimes including total body irradiation, are routinely used in large transplant centres, often employing the patient's own marrow to support them (see chapter 7). Early attempts to use this technique in small cell lung cancer were largely unsuccessful, but in breast cancer, preliminary data, mostly from the USA, really do look encouraging, suggesting a potential improvement in five-year survival figures for patients with high-risk disease. This is just the sort of example where a substantial multi-centre controlled clinical trial will be essential to see whether or not these exciting early data really translate into the improvements we all hope to see. One fascinating feature of this type of work is the way in which new ideas and technology spawn each other – for years, specialists have wished to deliver higher doses of chemotherapy, but have been prevented from doing so because of bone marrow suppression and other side-effects; now we have both the human growth factors, the CSFs referred to in the previous chapter, as well as the more powerful anti-nausea and other support methodology which allow us to at least ask the question with relative safety.

But one set of problems succeeds another. For instance, the myelo-suppression, or temporary bone marrow failure, following high-dose chemotherapy is substantially alleviated by the CSFs now widely available, but increasing the chemotherapy dose, say, threefold does inevitably bring different side-effects to the fore. So far we have not yet learnt how to cope with the severe skin reaction, gastro-intestinal toxicity, nerve damage (peripheral neuropathy) and, in some cases, temporary effects on the brain which some of the most useful drugs are likely to produce, if given in a high enough dose. It's no good dealing successfully with the neutropenia of bone marrow failure if the patient suffers severe exfoliation (peeling) of the skin instead, limiting the dose to a rather marginal fifty to a hundred per cent increase. It is worth repeating that, despite the remarkable effectiveness of CSF cytokines on stimulation and restoration of circulating blood levels, we do not as yet have any evidence that such treatment (often despite very considerable expense) saves more lives through a significantly improved anti-cancer effect of the higher dose chemotherapy.

Despite these many caveats, some recent approaches really have been valuable. High-dose chemotherapy, with support from autologous bone marrow transplantation (ABMT) or peripheral blood stem cells (PBSC), has already been referred to in chapter 7 and is clearly making waves in a variety of tumour sites. The increasing availability of PBSC support will undoubtedly widen the applicability of these techniques, since it is relatively simple to collect and concentrate the cells from circulating blood, so that several courses of chemotherapy can be safely dose elevated, rather than just the one, as tends to be the case with ABMT-supported therapy. Perhaps unexpectedly, some research teams have shown that the degree of bone marrow repopulation is even better with PBSC than with ABMT, a further bonus. The technique obviously has considerable promise in breast cancer, Hodgkin's disease, the non-Hodgkin lymphomas and refractory testicular tumours, in all of which the ABMT technique is either looking good or has already proven itself.

Infusional chemotherapy

Another interesting new idea is the use of infusional chemotherapy, again a means of delivering rather more chemotherapy in a given period of time (i.e. a second method for dose intensification). For some tumours, it already seems clear that this approach is more effective than with conventional chemotherapy – colorectal carcinoma appears to be a good example, and of particular interest, since traditionally (that is to say, up until about five years ago!) colorectal cancer was regarded as essentially insensitive to chemotherapy at all. Even now, many specialists would not regard these tumours as suitable cancers for chemotherapy treatment, though my view is that the evidence is now strongly against such a nihilistic judgement. Furthermore, by a curious piece of lateral thinking, we now know that folinic acid, a simple vitamin agent available in oral form and previously used only as an antidote to the antifolate drug methotrexate (introduced in 1948 – we've known about it for over forty years), has a quite different role in augmenting the effect of a quite different anti-cancer drug, 5-fluorouracil (see chapter 5), greatly enhancing its effect in these tumours. Apart from providing reasonably effective chemotherapy in this condition, perhaps for the first time, the use of constant infusion techniques, using a computerised pump attached to an implanted Hickman line (a cannula implanted through the skin, directed towards the heart and left in place for months if necessary) allows the patient to have the treatment at home. The infusion pump is secured in a holster or pouch, with only minimum interference from the usual day's work or leisure. This type of approach is being explored in many cancers and theoretically has advantages over the conventional, pulsed application of chemotherapy, since one might reasonably expect that tumour cells would have less opportunity to repair and regrow during the lengthy infusion period. It may also turn out, of course, that a constant infusion of CSF blood stimulators may be a highly effective means of preventing chemotherapy myelosuppression in the first place – perhaps making it still more possible to amplify dose in ways which we cannot consider at present. Higher doses of continuously infused chemotherapy drugs may represent a means of avoiding the non-myelosuppressive effects of these agents as well.

Interferons

A further exciting area which has also borne considerable fruit is the introduction of interferons – again, first considered something of a joke when initially introduced in the 1970s. Interferons (IFNs) are, strictly speaking, a group of agents that were first described as anti-viral in nature, but were investigated as possible anti-cancer drugs because of their cell killing (cytotoxic) effect, their ability to activate specific parts of the immune system and, finally, their relatively modest toxicity. Interferons are thought to work by stimulating or amplifying the immune system of the patient in such a way that 'rejection' of the cancer is rendered more likely; it also seems possible that the immune suppression, which may be a feature of 'successful' cancers (i.e. those which have taken hold and represent the greatest threat to the patient) could also be reversed.

Twenty years of research have demonstrated a definite role for interferons (chiefly interferon alpha) in a number of malignancies, including a rather unusual type of leukaemia known as 'hairy cell' leukaemia, because of the characteristic microscopic appearance of the cells; and another allied condition known as essential thrombocythaemia, a bone marrow condition in which there is over-proliferation of platelet precursors, leading to a dangerously high level of circulating platelets. In both of these disorders, interferon has established itself as the treatment of choice. Furthermore, recent data from several parts of the world, including Britain and the United States, have shown an impressive improvement in both response and survival rates in multiple myeloma, a fairly common,

incurable and often extremely painful condition (see chapter 23), characterised by proliferation of malignant plasma cells within the bone
marrow, and a whole host of clinical manifestations. In myeloma, the
benefit of interferon is more or less confined to patients who have
responded well to chemotherapy in the first place, but fortunately this
includes about seventy-five per cent of all patients with this condition.

The greatest interest in interferons at present lies in their possible
activity in some of the highly drug-resistant cancers we currently do so
poorly with, notably cancer of the kidney (renal cell carcinoma) and
malignant melanoma (the most feared of skin malignancies). In melanoma (see chapter 18), studies have addressed the issues of the best route
of administration and of the possible importance of high interferon
dosage. In one study, out of twenty-three patients with metastatic disease
probably incurable by other means, five objective responses were noted,
including three patients who had surprisingly durable complete remissions lasting more than two years. If substantiated, this would make
interferon a more effective form of systemic therapy than any currently
available type of anti-cancer chemotherapy, and a good deal less toxic. In
Kaposi's sarcoma, a serious skin malignancy common in young men with
AIDS, alpha interferon has delivered a reproducible response rate of
twenty to forty per cent, including some complete responses, in which all
signs of disease disappeared on therapy.

Interferon therapy is clearly still at an early phase of development.
There may genuinely be a worthwhile benefit in patients with solid
tumours, and it has also been claimed that interferon might enhance the
anti-tumour effects of radiation therapy whilst protecting normal tissues.
Although established only for a small number of rather unusual clinical
conditions, interferons could well turn out to be one of the more exciting
new therapies in the 1990s and beyond.

Radiation therapy: novel approaches

Although radiation therapy is now almost a hundred years old, there is
clearly much more to be learnt about its potential applications. We've only
just learnt how to use it as a systemic (i.e. whole-body) agent for total body

irradiation, and we're still not entirely sure of the safest method of dose delivery or the best dose compromise (between dangerous underdosage of the tumour and unnecessary side-effects from raising the dose too high) for all clinical conditions. In palliative work, which occupies about half of all we do, we've only recently learnt that reducing the number of treatment fractions, to the patient's considerable advantage and convenience, is just as effective as much more lengthy treatments. It also has the real benefit of freeing up departmental time so that lengthy radiation courses for other patients can be given more unhurriedly, in clinical situations which require such treatment. Radiation therapists are still looking for ways in which the benefit of the treatment can be increased by enhancing the differential cytotoxic effect on tumour and host tissue. One approach has been the use of radiosensitizer drugs, which the patient would take throughout a course of treatment (generally as a tablet by mouth), the idea being that this would sensitise the tissues in such a way that the radiation effect on the tumour would be greater than normal, without any corresponding effect on the host tissue cells. Unfortunately, despite considerable early promise and a few dramatic newspaper headlines, alas, none of the large-scale studies has yet shown benefit. There is nothing wrong with the idea, though.

One genuinely exciting area in radiation research is the use of hyperfractionated radiotherapy, i.e. the delivery of two or three fractions of treatment each day, rather than only one, with the total treatment time reduced from, say, six weeks to about two weeks. The advantages hoped for are not simply a matter of patient convenience, although reducing the total treatment by a month would obviously be an advantage. The hope is that such treatments will allow far less effective tumour cell recovery during treatment (particularly since the most ambitious of the treatment programmes treats patients seven days a week rather than five days per week, since theoretically the two-day gap at a weekend could allow for dangerous tumour recovery between conventional radiotherapy fractions given on a Friday and a Monday). At present, the Medical Research Council in the UK is supporting a large multi-centre randomised study comparing this approach (in two major sites: head and neck, and bronchus) to try and settle this issue. If the study turns out positive for the hyperfractionated group, the logistic consequences would, of course, be very profound.

Radiation and chemotherapy

Although not strictly speaking a new treatment any longer, the use of a combination of radiation and chemotherapy (increasingly popular and well researched over the past ten years or so) is clearly an approach which is set to continue and develop. It's an extremely logical form of therapy, combining the advantages of local irradiation for effective control of the primary tumour (either with conservative surgery, as in breast cancer, or no surgery whatsoever, as in many head and neck cancer cases) with the potential that chemotherapy has for eradication of metastatic disease. Increasingly, the trend is towards 'adjuvant' chemotherapy, in which the treatment is given so early – generally after completion of the primary local therapy (or even beforehand) shortly after the diagnosis is established – that there can be no certainty that the patient does indeed have even a microscopic degree of metastatic disease. The logic is, of course, based on the statistical probability that in certain types of patient – premenopausal breast cancer patients, for example, with positive lymph node involvement at the axilla – the risk of 'invisible' disseminated microscopic disease is very high indeed.

What has certainly become clear during the past few years is that, even with the relatively modest agents we currently have in tumours like breast cancer, early treatment at this stage offers the best possible opportunity for seriously damaging the microscopic metastases whilst the cell burden is small. All the evidence suggests that, even though breast cancer is incurable once established distant metastases become clinically identifiable, early 'adjuvant' treatment can be nonetheless successful, with clear-cut survival benefits demonstrable ten years after the relatively brief course of adjuvant chemotherapy was given. As an interesting digression, a large international group meeting in Oxford and representing the world's breast cancer experts, was asked in 1989 to predict these results, on the basis of the five-year results which had already been published. Not one of the distinguished company in that room got it right – about half felt the ten-year benefit would be more or less as it had been at five years, the other half (the pessimists) thinking that the benefit would have washed out altogether at the later observation date. In point of fact, the benefits at ten years are even greater than at five years (and the same is true for adjuvant tomoxifen) – which all goes to show that, however well informed you are, in medical science you can't trust your intuition – you have to do both the experiment and the follow up. I learnt a lot that day.

Adjuvant chemotherapy has also been shown to be beneficial in primary bone tumours and in locally advanced colorectal and possibly head and neck cancers. In the case of bone tumours, clinical management of the two major diseases (both tending to occur in adolescence) have been revolutionised by this treatment; in the case of head and neck and colorectal cancers, the benefit is clearly much more modest, but the numbers of patients far greater. In the childhood cancers, still the commonest natural cause of death in childhood (only accidents rate more highly), the whole situation has been transformed by adjuvant chemotherapy (see chapter 24).

There is no telling where it will all stop. I still remember the initial publications on adjuvant chemotherapy in 1976, less than twenty years ago, when we (the sceptical British, that is) on the whole took a rather disdainful view about the new claims, feeling certain that there must be alternative explanations for the 'apparent' benefits. But if adjuvant chemotherapy can reduce the death rate from breast cancer every year for the first ten years of follow up (and perhaps more, we don't yet know), there seems every reason to suppose that these survival improvements might possibly extend to other types of cancer too.

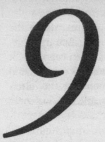

chapter nine

ALTERNATIVE THERAPIES AND THEIR LIMITATIONS

We all have our prejudices, I suppose, and one of mine, I freely admit, is a distaste for cure-all fashionable treatments whose claims are strongly advanced yet poorly supported by scientific evidence. Whoever first said, 'I've said it thrice, it must be true!' understood the power of speech, but doesn't get my vote.

I realise I'm on shaky ground when I attack the sacred cow of alternative remedies for cancer, but that, it seems to me, is what these remedies have become. Whilst not, I hope, too arrogant to accept that patients (and their oncologists) need all the help they can get, I have a deep suspicion of remedies whose advocates are reluctant to test them in the open court of prospective trials. Most of the few really well-designed studies that have been performed have turned out negative (or, worse still, suggested that the unconventional treatment might possibly do harm). There is also the potential problem that considerable sums of money can so easily be made from vulnerable, gullible and trusting victims. Of course, I recognise every cancer patient's wish not only to get well again, but better still to make a contribution to his or her own recovery. But devoutly wishing something were true doesn't, alas, make it happen, and in my experience, much harm, as well as the undoubted benefit from, say, a balanced, healthy diet, can be done by some of the unwise (but perhaps well-intentioned) suggestions that are made.

Patients with cancer may well decide to abandon medical treatment and opt for false or unproven remedies, such as extreme dietary manipulation, 'herbal' or 'natural' medicines, faith healing, visualisation therapy, shark-fin supplements, immunisations, intensive multi-vitamin additives and 'cleansing' coffee enemas. They may be urged to do so by relatives or other patients, sometimes adding these treatments to the conventional medicine, but often deciding that the two are incompatible, and that the conventional advice is no longer acceptable. Ten years ago, it seemed to me more common for alternative practitioners to recommend that patients should discard the conventional treatment for the 'alternative'. I believe this trend is now considerably less marked, a welcome step forward.

Patients who do abandon conventional treatment are often frightened or anxious, with strong ideas about the way their bodies work or what caused their cancer in the first place. They often believe strongly in 'bodily detoxification' – often after years of overindulgence. Sadly, however, even if dietary factors are important in causation, it is illogical to expect that the cancer will therefore be cured by an alteration in the diet or emotional attitude of the patient, or by taking up natural products, such as herbal remedies. However, the sad but incontrovertible truth is that giving up smoking does not cure lung cancer.

But what damage can these remedies do? Can it really be dangerous to attend a healing centre and experience the warmth, human love and goodwill that such places genuinely offer? What's so wrong with reflexology, iridology, coffee enemas, mega vitamin therapy or highly excluding diets? For a start, there is no evidence that any of these remedies work. No evidence of anti-tumour activity has ever been presented in a convincing way, no evaluation of results or independent critical assessment of data has been given. The anecdotes offered are on the lowest level of clinical value (see chapter 6) and are often explicable by simple means. Some cancer patients who profess to have been cured by unconventional remedies have, in fact, been following a conventional path as well, so any claim for the value of the alternative therapy is entirely clouded by a conventional treatment which is likely to have been responsible for the benefit. In one of the few controlled studies of alternative cancer treatment, laetrile, a 'harmless yet effective' remedy approved by most alternative cancer 'authorities' was found to be entirely without benefit and yet with significant side-effects when assessed in over 500 cancer patients treated at the Mayo Clinic. At least one major multicentre study carried out more recently has confirmed that other similar claims have no factual basis.

The process of mentally adjusting to a terrible diagnosis such as cancer can be badly shaken by false optimism, followed by despair at failure. It is cruel to raise false hopes, and one of my concerns about the term 'alternative therapy' is that it is in itself untruthful, when used to imply that a proven method of treatment is being offered. Worse still if the patient delays conventional treatment, sometimes with tragic consequences in the case of a potentially curable tumour. I have certainly seen this myself on a number of occasions, leading not only to personal tragedy, but terrible conflict if there is serious disagreement between family members as to the best way forward. Patients with advanced cancer can sometimes be cajoled or even bullied by their well-meaning relatives (generally of a younger generation) into taking an entirely 'natural' diet, then finding it intolerable and losing what remaining interest they may have had in nutrition. Despite considerable weight loss, they may even feel that they have to continue with the diet in order not to let their children down.

One of the many reasons that patients seek these remedies is a dissatisfaction with conventional medicine or with the doctor, which is a loss of faith and trust we must certainly take seriously. Doctors are certainly at fault – and must shoulder some of the responsibility – if patients cannot get sufficient of their time or reasonable answers to their questions. Patients often say that they tried alternative methods of treatment because they were given no hope or emotional support, because they found the prospect of radiotherapy or chemotherapy unnatural, because there was inadequate explanation and reassurance and because treatment was being unreasonably or thoughtlessly prolonged or aggressive, without any hint of benefit. If a patient does decide to discontinue treatment, against the advice of the specialists, it is, of course, only proper to advise the patient of what the consequences might be, but cruel to bully or browbeat the patient into continuing. The patient should at the very least be reassured that he or she would be welcome back at any later stage.

Despite these harsh words, I do, in fact, feel that it can be helpful to send a patient with cancer to a homeopath or other 'alternative' specialists. Many patients do have a mystical belief that a change of diet or lifestyle, or a visit to a herbalist or acupuncturist will generally be beneficial. I have considerable regard for the homeopathic physician I regularly send patients to (and who sends hers to me as well), partly because she can offer in a rational manner some of the things I cannot, and partly because she happens to be an excellent doctor with considerable rapport and communication skills. This seems to me to lie close to the heart of the appeal of alternative medicine and also, incidentally, to help explain why I don't any longer see the swell of patients asking for referral that were so much a feature of the 1980s. With the much greater use of counsellors within the health service, and a higher level of understanding among doctors of the importance of communication, it seems to me that the demand has considerably dwindled.

But for conventional medicine, there is another ever-present danger. As patient care becomes more and more technologically based, with patients passed from one specialist to another, there is often a real difficulty that a patient may lose sight of who is truly in charge of his case – who is at the apex of the pyramid, so to speak. When this happens, the stage is set for dissatisfaction and lack of confidence, though it seems to be one of the areas (ever decreasing, sadly) in which British medicine remains the best. Elsewhere, particularly in the USA, in which sub-specialisation is so common, many patients complain that they have to pinch themselves to remember quite who is in charge; our system may be technologically less highly tuned, but this particular mistake is, I believe, one we make less often.

So be on your guard against those who make powerful claims but can't support them. Most cancer specialists much prefer patients to bring their clinical faculties with them into the consulting room, and ask all the questions that are bothering them. But for heaven's sake, do the same thing when you are about to see an alternative practitioner. It is all too easy to assume that because mega vitamins, shark-fin supplements and trace elements are costly, they must be working!

10

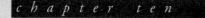

chapter ten

CONTINUING, TERMINAL AND HOSPICE CARE

F ew diseases are associated with such fear and anxiety as cancer, since so many of us assume that the disease will bring an inevitable progression of relentless new symptoms, uncontrollable suffering and certain death. One of the most difficult but rewarding tasks for the physician is to reassure patients that this is far from the truth, and to explain to him or her that cure or long-term remission is often possible. Although patients are better informed now than twenty years ago, partly as a result of wider discussion of cancer and its treatment within the media, medical knowledge, even among well-educated people, is often fragmentary and surprisingly incomplete. Although many patients may have recognised the seriousness of symptoms such as haemoptysis (coughing up blood) or a persistent swelling or glandular mass, many are unaware or, even if suspicious, too anxious to come forward to their general practitioner. Doctors, too, can be disinclined to speak frankly with patients, and some may not have the communication skills to do so. Specialists often fail to remember that even a condition such as breast cancer is not all that common in a general practice setting, compared with far more frequently encountered benign disorders.

For all these reasons, the importance of communication between specialists, patients and their general practitioners cannot be over-stressed. Indeed, communication is often the key to successful management of the most difficult problems of all, namely those in which cure is impossible and the outcome likely to be fatal. Specialists working in continuing and terminal care teams have frequently highlighted lack of communication, generally on the part of the specialist in charge, as the greatest barrier to satisfactory supportive care during the patient's final six weeks. They point out that a 'good' death is a realistic possibility, particularly since, during this final phase, when active treatment is no longer likely to be helpful, both the family and the patient are likely to have accepted the inevitable, at least in principle, perhaps to a greater degree than the doctors involved.

Continuing care

'Continuing care' is a loose term that is often taken to mean the care of a cancer patient who is unlikely to be cured, who is not yet close to death, but who has certain physical and emotional needs which are likely to be poorly served in the hospital setting, with its emphasis on acute and active care, action, noise, speedy recovery for others, and finally, a chronic lack of time for both medical and nursing staff to help the patient in the best possible way. For all these reasons, hospitals are increasingly regarded as far from an ideal setting for the care of cancer patients during the final weeks or months of life, quite apart from the economic cost of such expensive institutions remaining responsible for patients who, for the most part, don't need the high-tech services which have increasingly become the *raison d'être* for modern hospital in-patient care. Furthermore, incurable cancer patients traditionally received short shrift, until relatively recently regarded on some wards as patients beyond help, with correspondingly poor attention to their detailed needs, such as high-quality pain control, sympton relief (nausea, breathlessness, constipation and so on) and emotional support.

For all these reasons, the hospice movement, which developed twenty years ago, set out to provide special sanctuaries for patients like this who need a quite different environment – a calm setting instead of the usual ward buzz, with plenty of time for reflection and discussion with the staff, and a quite different set of priorities from that of the acute general hospital. The speed with which the movement took root is clearly an indication of the scale of the need, and Britain can certainly claim pride of place in the development of what has now become a world-wide attack on inadequate standards of care. One real benefit has been, ironically, that the hospital environment has also improved considerably over the past decade, with much more attention now being given to proper control of pain and other symptoms. Patients at most large hospitals no longer have to 'earn' their analgesic drugs (pain killers) in the way that used to be commonplace, not out of spite but generally the result of ignorance and an absurd misplaced fear, by doctors and nurses alike, of addiction to strong opiate drugs, such as morphine.

Increasingly, cancer patients, whether curable or not, are looked after in the community, often with the aid of Macmillan nurses (specially trained in cancer counselling, supportive care and generally highly skilled) or, better still, a multi-disciplinary team of individuals, often comprising nursing staff, social workers and one or more doctors, preferably with their own secretarial and administrative support. The development of these multi-disciplinary teams has resulted in far better care for cancer patients throughout the country than would have been dreamed possible even ten years ago, and most areas now have them. Financially, they make sense, since it is often possible to keep the patient at home – usually his or her preference anyway – where a hospital admission would otherwise be necessary. They are generally able to offer highly specialised advice about the appropriate choice and scheduling of pain drugs for cancer, and the prevention and treatment of side-effects both in active cancer treatment and in the palliative setting. Agents such as morphine can be quite difficult to handle. All strong pain killers, for example, tend to constipate, and it is extremely important for patients to be warned of this and to be given the appropriate laxative when starting opiates for the first time. This applies not only to morphine, but to all codeine derivatives (particularly the commonly used agent dihydrocodeine or DF118).

Multi-disciplinary teams can provide the best possible links between the specialist and the GP, generally visiting the patient as required, on a regular basis both at home and in hospital if the patient does require admission. Discussions between the team and members of the specialist oncology staff may well determine the most appropriate time for the patient's discharge, bearing in mind certain home needs, such as a modified bathroom with supportive rails and wheelchair access, or the transfer of a bedroom from an upper to a lower floor. Members of the support team are also likely to have built a closer relationship with family members than would have been possible in hospital, and may recognise better the key role of a spouse or partner in a patient's recovery, particularly if a major operation, such as mastectomy or radical hysterectomy has been necessary.

'HOW LONG HAVE I GOT?'

As recently pointed out by Dr Maurice Slevin, Chairman of the patient organisation BACUP (British Association of Cancer United Patients):

> *'It is almost always negative to tell people that they have a fixed life expectancy. The averages apply to populations and not to individuals, and to give people a fixed life expectancy removes hope and provokes depression and despondency. It is more appropriate and helpful to indicate that, while life might be very short if things go badly, the length of life could still be long and cannot be estimated if things go well'.*

The truth, of course, is that all of us, even specialists, are pretty imprecise when it comes to measuring the likely survival of a patient who cannot be cured. In this respect, medical predictions are generally wide of the mark, quite unlike what we have come to expect from watching too many Dr Kildare-style medical soaps. One recent study looking at this issue discovered that most doctors' predictions were too long, an expression, perhaps, of their innate optimism. Some patients, however, do feel they wish to be told a certain length of time, perhaps to put their affairs in order or to make a special trip, and this of course poses a particular difficulty for the doctor. It is usually better to provide an 'envelope' of time, rather than make a specific guess which is so likely to be wrong. It might seem a sensible idea to suggest a time interval which, on the face of it, is rather shorter than the doctor's genuine belief (partly on the grounds that patients gain considerable satisfaction from living longer than the doctor predicted), but this strikes me as a harsh approach, and, on the whole, I agree with Dr Slevin that it is better to express genuine uncertainty. One further problem comes with the strong request from a family member to be silent (or frankly mendacious), even if the patient him- or herself puts pointed questions about longevity. This really does put the doctor on the spot!

There is no easy answer to this difficult scenario. On the one hand, one might feel, as the doctor, that the family member – generally a husband or wife – has no right to place this constraint on the relationship that will have been built up with the patient, but on the other, the partner may have lived with the patient for twenty or thirty years and know him or her far better than the doctor can hope to. Ideally, one would prefer to respect this type of request, but frankly, at the end of the day, when there is a real conflict and the patient clearly wishes to have the doctor's most candid opinion, it seems to me that one's professional responsibility is to the patient above all others. Perhaps this is no different in principle from the situation discussed earlier in this book, namely the intrusive friend or family member who, at the first discussion with the professional, appears to be making all the running and asking questions which perhaps the patient would prefer not to voice him- or herself. On the other hand, the stakes are perhaps even higher, and certainly tensions more evident, where the question of life span is at issue, in a patient who is recognised by all parties as no longer being curable.

As Professor Souhami and I wrote in a medical textbook some years ago:

> ❧ *'There are few other branches of medicine which demand simultaneously such technical expertise and kindly understanding as does cancer medicine. The strains on the doctor are considerable, especially if he takes the human aspect of his work seriously. It is a great failing in a doctor if he talks to his patients only about the physical and technical aspects of the illness, relies heavily on investigation in making treatment decisions and finds it difficult to give up intensive measures and accept that the patient cannot be cured. Technical prowess is then replaced by thoughtful analysis of the patient's feelings and what is in his best interest.*
>
> *Treating patients with cancer demands great resources of emotional energy on the part of the doctor. In some units, part of the work of talking to patients is taken over by psychiatrists, psychologists, social workers or other counsellors. Invaluable though help from these persons may be, we do not think it desirable that doctors should see themselves as technical experts and that, when human feelings intrude into the medical situation, the patient should be sent to talk to someone else about their problems. Sustaining and counselling a patient and his relatives is a matter of teamwork, but the doctor in charge of the case must make it clear that he or she regards the psychological aspects of the disease to be as important as the physical.'* ❧

Pain and symptom control

The justifiable fear of unremitting pain as the cancer progresses, traditionally voiced by so many cancer patients in the past, should by now be unnecessary. We have a sufficient choice of versatile drugs for adequate pain relief to be possible in virtually all cases, although admittedly, considerable skill is required in order to achieve this. The use of regular, rather than 'as required', and appropriate medication, with laxatives, steroids, anti-depressants and so on, together with supportive drugs, has made an immense difference. Without wishing to appear too messianic, there really shouldn't be an excuse any longer for doctors to be over-cautious about increasing dosage, particularly of morphine, to the level required for adequate pain relief. One of the remarkable features of morphine as a pharmacological agent is its very wide spectrum of dose, probably wider than any other drug in use. Some patients require 30 milligrams twice daily of the commonly prescribed, long-acting morphine sulphate preparation, others ten times this or even more. The availability of the long-acting (twelve-hour) preparation has made patients' lives very much easier, since they no longer have to cart around large bottles of morphine elixir with them. The majority are now able to live comfortable and sometimes surprisingly normal lives, frequently continuing in this way – and deriving enormous psychological satisfaction from it – until shortly before death.

It's best to keep the pain prescriptions simple. For mild or moderate cancer pain, aspirin, paracetamol and co-proxamol (Distalgesic) are all helpful, and the first two, of course, can be purchased without a medical prescription. Anti-inflammatory agents, such as ibuprofen (now available in 200 milligram strength as Nurofen without prescription) are often also helpful in addition, though Nurofen is expensive and only half the strength of most medically prescribed tablets of ibuprofen (the commonest trade name for the 400 milligram strength is Brufen). Other useful drugs in this group are diclofenac (Voltarol) and naproxen (Naprosyn). For stronger pain relief, codeine and its derivatives are often prescribed, but are extremely constipating. This is such a demoralising and sometimes painful problem that it really is important to prevent it occurring in the first place. If the doctor doesn't prescribe you a laxative when offering codeine or dihydro-codeine for the first time, ask for one – you'll probably need it.

For severe or stubborn cancer pain, there really is no better drug than morphine. I have known countless patients who have been on lesser remedies for far too long before switching over; the sense of relief and improvement in their well-being is almost palpable. Many specialists prefer to start patients on the standard 10- or 20-milligram tablet given every four hours, since, before the days of long-acting morphine, it became increasingly well recognised that the duration of action of conventional morphine is limited to about four hours, so there is no earthly use in prescribing conventional morphine tablets or elixir at more extended time intervals than this. Starting a patient on morphine for the first time by using the four-hourly tablets does, of course, make sense from the point of view of flexibility, since at the early stage, it will be difficult to predict just what the dose requirement might be. Later on, however, it makes much more sense to switch to the long-acting, twelve-hourly tablets (known in the UK as MST and available in strengths of 10, 30, 60, 100 and 200 milligrams). A commonly used starting dose is 30 milligrams twice daily – 10 milligrams is generally too little. A few patients need to take the tablets every eight hours, presumably because of more rapid metabolism of the morphine than in the average case, but for most, the blood levels achieved by the twelve-hourly buffered preparation remain adequately high for the whole of that twelve-hour period. It is generally best to take the tablets at the same time night and morning, for example 8 p.m. and 8 a.m.

These long-acting morphine preparations have really revolutionised cancer care. Patients don't seem to need an inevitable increase in dosage anything like as quickly as might be imagined. Addiction simply isn't a problem, so the dose chosen should be whatever is required to give adequate pain relief, without going over the top, as it were. Many patients need the same dose night and morning, but in some patients, particularly those whose normal day is an active one, more MST might be required in the morning – say 60 milligrams, to help them through a busy twelve hours until 6 p.m. than the evening dose, which might remain at 30 milligrams. In my view, one of the greatest benefits of MST has been the enormous improvement in the quality of sleep, often for the first time after months of demoralising nocturnal discomfort.

There should rarely, if ever, be any need for regular intermittent morphine injections, but one very important route for powerful analgesia, in patients who can't take the tablets, is the subcutaneous infusion pump, which can be set up whilst the patient is still in hospital, or as an out-patient by a skilled nursing or medical support team, and continued more or less indefinitely, as required. The principle is that, using a fine butterfly needle implanted just under the skin, smooth delivery of pain killers (generally morphine or diamorphine) can be easily achieved, and other drugs added in as required, for nausea, for example. This is a system which is now commonly used and is perfectly compatible with a relatively normal life as an out-patient.

Above all else, it is never right for a doctor to shrug his or her shoulders and claim there is nothing more he or she can do. It is quite wrong to abandon the patient in this way; indeed, patients often make a far less clear-cut distinction between active and passive treatment than doctors do, and are generally extremely appreciative of the doctor's attempts to get the details of pain and symptom control right. It's not the gratitude that's important, of course, but the implication that to the patient these details really do matter. A good doctor should have skill, balance, judgement and compassion in equal measure, and it's every cancer patient's right to expect the best.

There can't, of course, be any simple solution to the best means of providing social support and symptomatic care during the final weeks or months of a patient's life. Individual circumstances vary so widely. But our increasing recognition that widespread cancer is not a diagnosis which needs to be stigmatised or pushed aside has helped immeasurably. So, too, has the wider application of the many principles of supportive care outlined above. With proper attention to detail, the right type of medication, adequate local resources and frequent review, either in the community or the follow-up clinic, many more patients can be helped so that 'death with dignity' becomes more than a hollow and unfulfilled promise.

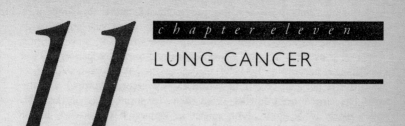

chapter eleven

LUNG CANCER

L ung cancer represents one of the greatest tragedies of the Western world, summed up, it seems to me, in the old *Punch* cartoon which showed Sir Walter Raleigh talking to his mate when they discover tobacco for the first time; the friend is saying, 'Well, don't worry, Walt; if we discover it's dangerous, we can always give it up.'

Causes of lung cancer

Lung cancer is by far the most common cancer in the West, having increased steadily in incidence since the 1930s. Cigarette smoking became popular in the trenches in the First World War, and we now know that the epidemic of lung cancer, wherever in the world you look at it, follows the introduction of cigarette smoking by about twenty years. This terrible fact is just as true for women, who started to take up smoking in large numbers in the 1950s, just as men did thirty years before. The relationship between cigarette smoking and lung cancer is absolutely clear cut, and we also know that stopping smoking is most certainly followed by a reduction in the individual's risk of developing lung cancer. After about fifteen years of non-smoking, the risk is almost as low as if the individual had never smoked at all, an observation very clearly shown in a long-term study of British doctors who, as a group, rapidly cut down their smoking in the 1960s after the link had been established, and were later found to be at very much reduced risk of lung cancer than before.

It is tragic that so many young people smoke, and there is no doubt that the tobacco industry has substantially targeted this group, with considerable success. In the 1950s, the male-to-female ratio for lung cancer was over ten to one, i.e. women formed under ten per cent of the total lung cancer group. By 1984, the figure stood at only four to one (i.e. twenty-five per cent of all lung cancer cases were now women), and the gap has closed even further since then. In some parts of the UK, particularly in Scotland, lung cancer in women has overtaken breast cancer as the commonest of all female cancers.

Recent debate has centred on the dangers of passive smoking, and it is now known that non-smoking women who are married to smokers face a risk of lung cancer which is over twice what it would be if they (as non-smokers) were married to men who also did not smoke. The Royal College of Physicians has just issued a devastating report on the dangers of passive smoking in children, including the probability of an increased risk of cot death, asthma and other childhood diseases. In Britain, cigarettes are now relatively cheaper than they were twenty-five years ago, and restriction of smoking in public areas has been a protracted and uphill battle. There is now a clear and inverse relationship, both in Britain and the United States, between social class and the incidence of lung cancer, which seems entirely attributable to smoking, since social classes 1 and 2 have a much lower rate than social classes 4 and 5. Moreover, the death rate from this disease is extremely high, since it is both common and, in most cases, very difficult to cure.

Other causes of lung cancer pale into insignificance when compared to cigarette smoking, at least in the Western world, where industrial pollution and radiation exposure is, for the most part, not such a major issue. In the Middle and Far East, and other areas of the developing world, lung cancer is emerging as a major health hazard, just as in the West. These countries face an uphill struggle against the self-promotion of a powerful and sophisticated tobacco industry, unrestrained by the governmental and social pressures which now operate, at least in part, in the West.

That is not to say that there are grounds for complacency here at home. Although a no-smoking policy now operates in many public places, on public transport and so on, the rates of incidence and mortality from lung cancer are falling only slowly, and, in some social groups, barely at all. There is no proof as yet that low-tar brands, now very actively advertised, are necessarily safer than traditional ones, or that the government health warnings we see on hoardings and cigarette packs are all that effective. One brand of cigarettes even promotes its macho image by exploiting the links between smoking and fatal cancer, cynically justifying its advertising by donating a small part of the profit to fund research. Many believe that a total ban on tobacco advertising would be far preferable; I count myself among them. Children and young people can all too easily obtain cigarettes and fall prey to a disgusting habit which will dent their finances, clog their heart and lungs, stain their teeth, make them and their clothes smelly and unappealing, and, in the end, quite possibly prove fatal. The cost of treating cigarette-related diseases (the cost to all of us, that is, since most of us are tax payers) is enormous, particularly since chronic heart and lung disease may persist for years before the death of the patient. If cigarette smoking had never been invented, so to speak, our commonest cancer would be something of a medical rarity, and individual cases would be written up as medical curiosities in the professional journals.

Instead of which, we have an epidemic of horrendous proportions. Patients who smoke between ten and twenty cigarettes a day have a risk of lung cancer which is thirty times greater than those who do not smoke at all; for people who smoke more than forty cigarettes a day, the risk is well over sixty times greater. Well over 30,000 people in Britain develop lung cancer each year, the majority of whom die from it, usually within two years of diagnosis. Many of these patients are in their fifties and sixties. Of the other risk factors for lung cancer, only asbestos and air pollution are seriously worth considering, though these are far less important. Since lung cancer is such a difficult type of tumour to cure, and so damaging in its effects before death, the importance of cutting down, or, better still, stopping smoking cannot be overstressed. Paradoxically, though, patients who have spent a lifetime smoking, and then develop lung cancer, are the one group who seem to stop smoking, when it is, of course, far too late. Sometimes, when I have seen the third or fourth new lung cancer patient at the clinic, I feel a sense of despair as the patient tells me, 'No Doc, not at all,' in response to my standard 'What about smoking?' question, only to reply lamely, 'About three weeks ago,' when asked how long it's been since he stopped. The previous forty years at twenty a day seem to have been forgotten.

People do have a perfect right, of course, to self-destruct as they think fit; it is not for me to preach. (Although with the growing proof of the effects of passive smoking, there is always the health of those around to consider.) However, I do think it is important that patients realise that stopping smoking when a cancer is diagnosed isn't all that likely to prove beneficial and certainly won't make the cancer go away. The only time to do it is Now! If patients just diagnosed with lung cancer do find it difficult to stop, I don't think it's right to press them all that hard since, to be blunt, the majority will not survive anyway. On the other hand, there is a small group, those who do well with treatment, who most certainly should be urged to stop, since, most tragically, further smoking might induce a second cancer which could prove to be the fatal one. This is certainly the case in patients who have had successful treatment of a cancer of the larynx (see chapter 2) – itself a smoking-induced cancer in many cases. Early treatment of these laryngeal tumours is so successful that the commonest cause of death is a lung cancer from continued smoking!

Types of lung cancer

There are many types of lung cancer. The commonest is a typical squamous cell carcinoma (see chapter 3), one of the common tumour types which arise from the lining of the lung passages, usually one of the main bronchi, the major pathway from the trachea, or windpipe, to the lungs themselves. This type of tumour accounts for over half of the cases we see in Britain and is exceptionally rare in non-smokers. This also applies to another important tumour type, the small cell lung cancer, which pathologically and in its natural history is a quite different entity. It may look the same on a chest X-ray, but, in reality, the small cell variety of lung cancer is even more lethal, with very rapid spread to other parts of the body, and a high rate of malignant cell division, making it the most rapidly fatal of all the lung cancers, with a very poor cure rate, despite initial response to treatment (see below). This, too, is particularly closely associated with cigarette smoking, unlike the less common variety of lung cancer, the adenocarcinoma (see chapter 3), which would probably be the commonest type of lung tumour if cigarette smoking were not so common.

Squamous cell and adenocarcinoma, together with a third type known as the large cell carcinomas, form a group often referred to as 'non-small cell lung cancer' to distinguish them from the small cell variety. They are often lumped together in this way, since the treatment policies are similar for each and quite different from what we recommend for small cell lung cancer. This is discussed in more detail below.

Symptoms and diagnosis

Typical symptoms in lung cancer patients include coughing, often with bloodstained sputum, shortness of breath and chest pain. Many patients will be used to these symptoms, since smokers frequently develop chronic bronchitis and come to expect winter exacerbations. However, in patients with lung cancer, the symptoms are often more severe, and the sputum may be bloodstained for the first time. Some patients develop a pneumonia which is slow to resolve despite antibiotics, and some with difficulties in swallowing because of the compression of the oesophagus (gullet) caused by enlarged cancerous glands in the chest. Many have weight loss, having become increasingly uninterested in food; others will turn up for the first time, not with symptoms relating to the primary tumour, but, bearing in mind the frequency with which lung cancers spread to other parts of the body, with symptoms from this secondary spread. This might include, for example, severe pain or even a fracture of a long bone or vertebra from a secondary bone deposit; sudden loss of function of an arm or leg from a secondary deposit (often multiple) in the brain; or the patient may have noticed an enlarged gland in the neck, which, on biopsy, turn out to be an obvious site of secondary tumour spread.

Diagnosis is usually straightforward. Most lung cancers are easily visible on a chest X-ray, and confirmation of an abnormal shadow can usually be obtained either by examination of sputum under the microscope ('sputum cytology') or by a technique known as broncho-scopy, in which a semi-flexible fibre-optic tube is passed, under a light anaesthetic, through the nose, larynx and trachea, down the bronchial tube, to the site of the abnormality, which is usually pretty obvious from the X-ray. The physician can then take a small biopsy under direct vision – in most cases of lung cancer, the malignant ulcer will be easily visible. Occasionally, particularly in elderly or infirm patients, one has to accept an X-ray without further biopsy as being sufficient for diagnostic purposes, but by and large, as with all other cancers, specialists increas-ingly (and rightly) take the view that a label marked 'cancer' should not be hung around the patient's neck until a firm pathological diagnosis has been made.

Lung cancers are amongst the most dangerous and lethal of all, since they can spread so widely – particularly the small cell variety. Potential secondary sites include liver, brain, long bones and vertebrae, skin, lymph nodes and intra-abdominal soft tissues – almost anywhere, in fact. For these reasons, surgical removal of a lung cancer, so valuable in a minority of patients, cannot always be relied upon.

Treatment

Which brings us to treatment. There is no doubt that, wherever possible, a lung cancer should be surgically removed, since this technique has the greatest chance of long-term success. The trouble is that only a smallish minority of lung cancer cases are really suitable for surgery. In the first place, all the small cell lung cancer cases (about twenty-five per cent of the total) are surgically out of bounds, since they are very likely to have spread beyond the primary site to one of the more distant areas. This is generally accepted to be the case, even where exhaustive scanning and other staging investigations have failed to reveal secondary deposits outside the chest. Surgery for these patients just makes things worse, apart from a tiny minority with peripherally placed small accessible tumours – and even in this group, there is considerable doubt as to whether surgery, though technically possible, is really worth pursuing.

In the non-small cell cancer group, surgery is worth considering, but will only be recommended if the patient fulfils certain criteria. The tumour must not be situated too close to the centre of the chest, for example, since the closer it lies to the point of division of the two main bronchi from the windpipe (the carina), the less possible it will be for the surgeon to clear the tumour, even if he is prepared to remove the whole of one lung (pneumonectomy). The more peripherally placed the tumour, the more operable it will be, and all surgeons (and all patients) would prefer to simply perform a lobectomy (removal of part of the lung, the lobe in which the tumour is situated) than remove the whole lung itself. The functional consequences are far less severe. The general condition of the patient must, of course, be adequate, an important point, since many have been heavy smokers in the past, and may therefore be suffering from other conditions, such as bronchitis or heart disease, which will render them unsuitable for surgery, even if, by other criteria, they have an operable tumour. Some patients have a collection of fluid below the lung which is likely to contain malignant cells (a malignant plural effusion), which again counts against them as far as operability is concerned, since the surgeon knows that these patients have an unacceptable probability of local tumour occurrence after surgery. And so on.

For patients with non-small cell lung cancer who are inoperable for any of these reasons, radiotherapy is worth considering, but in truth is likely to be most valuable as a means of palliation of symptoms, rather than as a treatment offered with any real prospect of cure. For symptoms such as coughing up blood, chest pain, obstruction of a large-bore bronchial pathway or swallowing difficulty from nodal enlargement, radiotherapy may be extremely valuable, but there is no point in taxing the patient with a very high dose of radiotherapy in the hope of cure, since a cure cannot be achieved except very rarely, with the exception of patients who fulfil all of the criteria for operability, but either turn down an operation (some do, surprisingly) or have another serious condition which makes the anaesthetic too risky.

There are particular situations where radiotherapy can be really valuable. As a result of direct pressure from the cancer, some patients develop a life-threatening degree of obstruction of the main blood vessel (superior vena cava) which returns blood from the upper half of the body. This syndrome of superior vena cava obstruction can cause tremendous pressure in the face and neck, with a bloated, bluish appearance and strikingly visible distended veins in the neck. Although rapidly fatal if left untreated, radiotherapy often provides quick and quite effective relief. Complete collapse of a lung may occur again as a result of direct pressure from the primary tumour or enlarged glands. Radiotherapy can shrink these masses, sometimes to the point of re-inflating the lung again. Other important clinical syndromes in lung cancer include loss of voice from erosion of the laryngeal nerve by a tumour mass deep in the chest, or destruction of the upper part of the chest wall and ribs (often with severe shoulder pain and weakness of the arm) by a tumour situated at the lung apex ('Pancoast syndrome'). For this latter indication, surgery can also be extremely valuable, though it may have to be quite radical. For tumours which have eroded the laryngeal nerve, surgery is not generally possible.

In small cell lung cancer, the treatment is altogether different because surgery is never sufficient (and is therefore not worth doing at all), and both chemotherapy and radiation are more appropriate. Most patients with small cell cancer respond to chemotherapy in the first instance, often to a striking degree, though to the clinician, this is one of the most frustrating of all tumours, since the early response to chemotherapy, often remarkable and able to produce a normal chest X-ray once again, is rarely maintained, as most patients develop drug resistance, often within a year or two of the initial treatment. It is not uncommon to share with the patient the joy of seeing the chest X-ray return to normal, only to point out grimly, perhaps six months later, the equally clear evidence of the return of the cancer – with inevitably fatal consequences.

There is no clear advantage for one type of chemotherapy over another. Over the years, my own hospital and other groups have tried to improve the chemotherapy effect by increasing the dose, adding additional agents, winding up the frequency of chemotherapy courses to the maximum possible level or even by introducing new experimental agents. None of these approaches has proved markedly superior to our previous attempts, but one recent improvement, at least for patients with 'limited disease', i.e. a tumour confined to the chest, without any evidence of spread, has been the use of combined chemotherapy and radiotherapy to the chest, a treatment approach now known to be more beneficial (but not dramatically so, it has to be said) than the use of chemotherapy alone. It's more taxing too, with side-effects such as swallowing difficulty from inflammation of the oesophagus (oesophagitis) and skin discomfort within the irradiated area. Radiotherapy alone, without chemotherapy, is rarely used for small cell lung cancer (apart from patients who are felt to be too unwell to cope with chemotherapy), since the therapeutic approach is obviously confined to the chest itself and would miss any opportunity for treatment of secondary tumours at other sites.

The outlook in lung cancer is generally poor. Patients who are suitable for a surgical removal of the tumour are in a fortunate minority group, and some surgeons claim cure rates in as many as fifty per cent of such cases. Sadly, however, these are very much the minority overall, and hardly any other patients with lung cancer are curable, apart from a small group with small cell lung cancer (ten per cent at the most) who respond dramatically and durably to chemotherapy, and patients with non-small cell lung cancer who very occasionally do well, long term, with radical radiotherapy. In small cell lung cancer, the frustrating paradox is that this tumour is so readily responsive to chemotherapy, at least in the first instance, yet overall has the worst outlook of any lung cancer type, with a very poor secondary response to chemotherapy (i.e. on relapse) despite the initial benefits that chemotherapy achieves. In non-small cell lung cancer, although chemotherapy has no traditional role, there are preliminary indications from recent studies that chemotherapy may turn out to have a modestly beneficial role after all. Once again, British trial groups (and others) are trying as best they can to pursue randomised studies, which are the only means of settling this question for sure.

For patients with secondary spread from a lung cancer, radiotherapy is once again the most valuable form of treatment, particularly in patients with bone metastases. This is equally true for the small cell and non-small cell varieties.

Case histories

MARY'S STORY

Mary had always been a heavy smoker – she admitted to forty a day, but I knew from her husband it was nearer sixty. She was fifty-four and worked as a barmaid in the local pub round the corner from the hospital; she had known most of the medical staff since they were students. 'I could tell you a few stories about him, for a start,' she'd say, pointing to my registrar.

She was brought into casualty suddenly, severely breathless and with a handkerchief full of blood clot. She'd been lying low for a bit, she said, but knew something was probably wrong when her heart started racing and she'd not been able to calm herself with the first cigarette of the day. Like so many patients with lung cancer, she'd suddenly gone off cigarettes entirely after smoking, I suppose, about a quarter of a million of them during her lifetime.

The chest X-ray showed complete collapse of the right lung, so no wonder she was breathless. The chest team did the bronchoscopy and saw a large tumour sitting only 2 centimetres away from the carina – the bifurcation of the trachea (windpipe) into the right and left main bronchi. 'I don't suppose all that smoky atmosphere in the pub helped one bit, Doctor,' said her husband.

It turned out to be a small cell cancer, best treated by chemotherapy. She was treated within one of our prospective trials, receiving six courses of chemotherapy and a month of radiation therapy to the chest. Although it never returned to normal, the chest X-ray dramatically improved, and her lung reinflated. There was champagne the night she returned to the bar.

Four months later, a gland appeared in her neck. A needle biopsy confirmed the worst. 'How could it have come back so fast, Doctor?' asked her husband. Like most patients with small cell lung cancer, Mary's tumour, though so responsive the first time round, proved almost fully resistant to chemotherapy on the second occasion. After two courses of chemotherapy using newer drugs not included in the initial choice, it was clear that we were getting nowhere. Local radiotherapy to the neck was successful in shrinking down the glandular mass, but within a further two months, she had developed secondary deposits in the liver, ribs and skin. 'Surely there must be something more that you can do?' said her husband. Sadly, there wasn't.

Small cell lung cancer has a very poor prognosis, all the more tragic since it is so closely related to cigarette smoking and would be a rare condition if smoking had never been invented, so to speak. However, not all patients with lung cancer do so poorly. Patients with operable cancers (always of the non-small cell variety) have a real chance of cure.

ERIC'S STORY

Eric, a retired seventy-four-year-old stockbroker who had stopped smoking ten years before I met him, initially saw his doctor because of mild shortness of breath and discomfort across the front of the chest. An X-ray showed a 4-centimetre tumour in the left upper lobe with a small cavity within; CT scanning showed no evidence of glandular involvement in the centre of the chest. His general condition was pretty good, so the local chest physician sent him to a thoracic surgeon, who performed his usual pre-operative investigation of walking together with the patient up three flights of stairs; he noted that Eric was no more out of breath than he was, and decided that he was fit for surgery. Four years later, after a left upper lobectomy (with preservation of about half of the left lung, leaving the right side untouched), the patient remains well and is probably out of the woods. Even though Eric developed lung cancer from lifelong cigarette smoking, he did himself a great favour by giving up, even at the late age of sixty-four. The other good thing about him is that he's now become a fanatic fund-raiser for cancer charities.

12

BREAST CANCER

B reast cancer has reached almost epidemic proportions in the Western world, with well over 20,000 new cases occurring annually in England and Wales alone. We have the dubious privilege of being the nation with one of the highest incidence rates in the world, and in British women, breast cancer is the commonest cancer (both in incidence and also in overall deaths from malignant disease). Media interest has never been higher, hardly a week going by without news of a new treatment, an unexpected risk from an established therapeutic approach, the uncertain benefits of routine mammographic scanning and so on. Many books have been written on this topic alone, and research into breast cancer has never been more active or better financially supported. Yet progress is agonisingly slow, with unsubstantiated or false claims about treatment breakthroughs far more common than genuine advances.

At least one in ten of Western women will develop the disease during their lifetime; three-quarters of these will be patients in the post-menopausal period of life, i.e. over the age of fifty, and it's in this group that mammographic screening appears to produce the greatest benefit. The principle, of course, is that small tumours, so small that they may be impossible to feel, can nonetheless be detected by mammography and therefore be more successfully treated than larger tumours, with, at the end of the day, a better chance of survival. A further important part of the rationale for mammographic screening in this group is that the disease is so common in the unselected female population that the pick-up rate will be high enough to justify both the expense and the anxiety caused by the call back for further testing or biopsy of a patient who might turn out, in fact, to have a benign breast disorder – also an extremely common phenomenon in the Western world, indeed far more so than breast cancer itself. It is not enough simply to state in a research publication that so many cases of cancer have been picked up and treated earlier than otherwise would have been possible; this important but inconclusive observation does not in itself prove that the whole endeavour is necessarily worthwhile. We need to know that earlier treatment of screen-detected cancers really does lead to better survival. Patients who are screened regularly but develop breast cancer in the period between these screenings (so called 'interval cases') often feel extremely angry that nothing was picked up.

The latest research (published in the *British Medical Journal* in January 1995) strongly suggests that the current recommendation of three years between screening mammography tests will fail to pick up substantial numbers of these cases.

Causes of breast cancer

We know quite a lot about the causation of breast cancer. It is clearly a disease in which a family history is important, and women with a first-degree relative with breast cancer have a threefold increase in risk. The more relatives, the higher the risk, particularly where the relative developed the tumour herself at a young age. We also know that women who have no children, or who have their first pregnancy after the age of thirty, are about three times more likely to develop breast cancer than those who are twenty or younger, the risk also increases with a late menopause or early age when the periods first start. Data from Hiroshima point quite clearly to radiation being a cause, though one fascinating feature of the biological studies following the atomic bomb survivors is that it took far longer to recognise breast cancer as being increased in incidence (about thirty-five years) than with other types of radiation-induced tumour also caused by the bomb.

Patients often ask how long they have had the breast cancer for, and it's never really possible to say, since all cancers are thought to begin with mutation of a single cell, well before any possibility of recognition by any known method. Some are even genetically predetermined, probably by a particular gene sequence in affected individuals. Since we know that it took thirty-five years for a slight but real statistical increase in the number of women developing breast cancer after the radiation blast to show up, we must assume, I think, that most breast cancers start their development many years (probably decades) before they make their visible or palpable appearance. Interestingly, one of my patients, who has absolutely no family history of breast cancer, told me that she and her sister, both in their forties, both developed breast cancer within a single year of each other and had both, during their teens, received annual chest X-rays (at a time when their breasts would have been developing) since their father had suffered from tuberculosis, and annual chest X-ray screening was frequently performed in those days. I found this rather a compelling story, particularly since the time interval was again thirty years.

There are certainly wide differences in incidence across the world – high in Europe and North America, low in many parts of Asia and Africa. In Britain, the overall incidence is clearly rising, with an eleven per cent increase noted between 1968 and 1978. My own belief is that this will continue since, with changing social patterns, better obstetrics and more efficient methods of contraception, women are putting off the age of their first pregnancy until later and later. Earlier this year, it was announced that the mean age of first pregnancy is now twenty-eight years – surely a decade or so beyond the physiological norm. Don't get me wrong; I'm not making a judgement about right and wrong, simply stating what I believe is a likely interpretation of a most unpalatable public health problem.

Symptoms and diagnosis

Almost all breast cancers arise from the glandular lining of the milk forming ducts and their tributaries, in other words they are typical adenocarcinomas (see chapter 3). True invasive breast cancer is easy to recognise pathologically (in a surgical biopsy specimen) because the so-called basement membrane of the duct will have been breached as the tumour cells spill into the deeper tissues of the breast itself. Non-invasive, or intraduct, breast cancer is also well recognised, though the two conditions can co-exist. It can occur multi-focally – at several sites – within the breast, so a single biopsy specimen, even if it shows no evidence of invasive disease, may not be adequate to exclude invasive breast cancer in other parts of the breast.

Although the Forrest recommendations for frequency and age group for screening are quite specific, there are clearly patients who ought to be examined mammographically more frequently, though it is difficult to be more specific. The higher the risk, the more reasonable it is to start screening at an earlier age. In an extreme example, one might envisage a young woman of thirty-five, with no children herself and a very strong family history of breast cancer, including an identical twin sister who, out of the blue, revealed that she had developed breast cancer three years beforehand, but had not told her twin for fear of upsetting her. Obviously a patient like this should be screened without delay, and then again at – what? – yearly intervals? Some might even suggest more frequently than this. In the USA, this is the kind of patient who might well be offered a subcutaneous mastectomy, i.e. removal of all the breast tissue but with preservation of the skin and nipple, with immediate surgical reconstruction. As is the case so often, what happens in the States today takes off in Britain tomorrow (though sometimes it is the other way round!), and more and more British surgeons feel that this kind of approach may have a place in highly selected patients.

Apart from patients who present through screening programmes, the main symptomatic group – still the majority – usually come to their GPs with a lump in the breast which either they or their partner has felt. Most women know enough about breast cancer to realise that the sooner they seek medical advice, the better. No doctor will mind being consulted for a breast lump that is quite obviously something other than cancer, or even for a breast lump which might be of the 'here today, gone tomorrow' variety – they do exist, since a benign breast disorder may wax and wane with the periods. Some patients know their breasts intimately, some not; some have had so much trouble over the years with cysts, recurrent breast pain, benign breast problem of one type or another that they live in constant fear of developing breast cancer and bring any new finding to their doctor's attention without delay. The other, more laid back type of patient may be just as liable, though, to develop the illness and by far the most sensible advice must be 'show any breast lump to the doctor and let him or her decide what's to be done'.

There is a ten to one chance that it is benign. This is a fairly consistent figure emanating from many breast cancer clinics up and down the country, and I hope that women will find it reassuring. Even a specialist surgeon may feel it is impossible to be certain of the nature of a lump, even after a thorough examination, without at the very least a mammogram, possibly even a biopsy. Mammograms are pretty safe nowadays, with a far lower risk of radiation exposure than previously, and no apparent danger, as far as one can tell, even when repeated on a regular basis every two years or so. This may seem inconsistent with my story of the two sisters with breast cancer, but many believe (myself among them) that it is the timing which matters, the developing breast of a young teenage girl being far more sensitive from the carcinogenic (cancer risk) point of view than the mature breast – and anyway, a mammogram now delivers less radiation than a chest X-ray.

How does a breast cancer feel? Usually the lump is fairly firm, often situated quite close to the nipple and most typically in the upper outer quadrant of the breast rather than the lower part or the inner portion. Most breast cancers are painless but slightly tender when pressed or squeezed. Nipple discharge is unusual, unless the cancer actually involves the area just behind the nipple itself. The skin is generally normal in appearance, but a cancer situated close to the surface can distort the skin, producing a characteristically dimpled appearance, sometimes particularly evident when the patient leans forward and the breast hangs more freely. If there are obvious glands in the axilla (armpit), this is further evidence that the lump could well be malignant. The rest of the breast – away from the lump – and the other breast generally feel completely normal. If there is an ulcer, i.e. the surface of the skin is broken, this also is an important visible sign of possible cancer, and the same applies to an obvious elevation of the area of skin corresponding to the lump. Do not delay! See the doctor, and then you will know one way or the other. Patients with tender, painful breasts, particularly when the cycle of discomfort corresponds to the menstrual periods, can almost always be reassured that the cause is benign.

Confirmation of the diagnosis is usually performed as an out-patient by the surgeon in the breast clinic, who will be the first port of call after referral from the family doctor. In the bad old days, patients were often subjected to what is now regarded as a pretty barbaric approach: 'We'll put you under an anaesthetic, remove the lump, and, if immediate examination confirms it is cancer, we'll perform a mastectomy there and then.' This approach has, thankfully, been pretty much abandoned now, and patients are far more frequently treated with greater compassion, and the diagnosis confirmed (or excluded) by fine needle aspiration of the breast lump, performed as an out-patient. This involves a simple procedure whereby the surgeon (or sometimes an expert pathologist) inserts a fine needle and syringe combination, just as for breast cysts, sucking gently in order to produce a tiny volume of material which can immediately be smeared onto a microscope slide. This simple technique (though it does take skill, and a certain knack, to get the most consistent results) gives plenty of cells spread out thinly in such a way that diagnosis of a malignant tumour or benign disorder can generally be made with complete confidence, though occasionally the test may have to be repeated if the initial result is equivocal.

Treatment

BREAST PRESERVATION OR MASTECTOMY?

If the aspiration test confirms cancer, the next step is to decide on the appropriate operation. Twenty years ago, this was a simple matter – patients were treated by mastectomy, the more radical the better. However, during the period since I qualified as a doctor (1971), there has been a complete rethink about this. We now have excellent evidence from several large studies that local excision ('lumpectomy'), together with post-operative radiotherapy in many cases (there are always exceptions, as I will show) gives results at least as good as mastectomy. For the most part, the preserved breast looks excellent, has a normal nipple, with a natural feel to it and no loss of sensation. In the majority of cases, no surgical reconstruction will be necessary. For all these reasons, more and more surgeons are happy to restrict the surgical removal to a lumpectomy, generally combined with an axillary node dissection in order to remove the whole of the lymph nodes in the axilla, to achieve both surgical control (so that the radiotherapist does not have to give radiotherapy to the armpit area) and also to provide the best possible information about the presence or absence of lymph-node involvement by the tumour. This is extremely important, since this feature of breast cancer provides the clearest indicator as to the likely outcome. Patients with small primary tumours, for example, and no evidence of involvement in a good sample of twenty or so axillary lymph nodes have a good outcome and are quite difficult to distinguish statistically from the normal population, at least for the first ten years after diagnosis and treatment. On the other hand, in a young woman with a large primary tumour and heavy axillary lymph node involvement, the outcome is much less satisfactory and further treatment with chemotherapy, hormone therapy or both should be given (more about this later).

Some patients are, however, better treated by mastectomy than breast preservation. First of all, there are patients with relatively large but still operable tumours in a small breast, in whom an attempt at lumpectomy would produce a very misshapen and cosmetically unsatisfactory result. Far better to do a simple mastectomy, possibly with primary breast reconstruction or – to many patients' satisfaction – the use of an external prosthesis. Second, there are certain patients who prefer to undergo mastectomy, feeling rightly or wrongly that they would sooner go the whole hog in order to be as safe as possible. It would be quite wrong to bully these patients away from a firmly held view, even if technically the lumpectomy procedure were possible. Finally, patients with a centrally placed tumour, just behind the nipple, may sometimes be better off with a mastectomy since local excision would require removal of the nipple, a serious cosmetic, sexual and emotional loss, though this is very much a matter for discussion between the surgeon and the patient (and perhaps the patient's partner as well, if she wishes). Finally, it is well worth remembering that, for all the advantages of a preserved breast, the necessary post-operative radiotherapy can be arduous and can never be accomplished as quickly as a mastectomy, so elderly or frail patients may be better treated by mastectomy, if they do not object to the operation. This will spare them the inconvenience of radiotherapy, particularly if they happen to live far from an oncology centre and do not have a strong preference for breast-preserving treatment. Patients don't all have the same priorities when it comes to sense of body image, concerns about intimacy and sexuality, etc.

RADIOTHERAPY

Not all specialists would agree that a course of radiotherapy is essential, even in patients who have been treated by lumpectomy alone, though the traditional view (which I share) is that the risk of local recurrence following lumpectomy alone is so high – at least forty per cent – that it is hard to see how radiotherapy can be avoided, even though I agree that a local recurrence within the breast is not a life-threatening event. You could argue, I suppose, that further surgery and/or radiotherapy could always be given to these self-selected cases, whilst other patients had got away with less treatment and therefore less risk of side-effects. But I do feel, however, that any recurrent event in breast cancer is best avoided, and most specialists endorse this general view; there is even evidence that a local recurrence may, to some extent, predict a more generalised recurrence, which, of course, is a far more significant and serious event.

There is no firm agreement on the specifics of the post-operative radio-therapy, some centres preferring a relatively short course, in the region of three weeks, whilst others go more slowly, taking the treatment over six weeks and with a lower radiation dose per day. Some regard this as an appalling and unjustifiable medical failing, arguing forcefully that we should all be far more consistent and cannot all be doing it right! My own view is that this type of difference (in technical detail) is quite typical of many situations in medicine, where specialists offer an approach which is likely to be coloured by all sorts of influences, including their own training, philosophy and the resources available to them. Although I'm well aware that some patients treated by radiotherapy for breast cancer do develop side-effects at a later stage (those with serious problems are fortunately a very tiny proportion of the numbers we treat), there doesn't seem to be any clear evidence that patients undergoing a rapid, three-week treatment course have more to fear from long-term side-effects than those who are treated at a slower rate over six weeks. I'll have more to say about the long-term side-effects of radiotherapy (including the allegations following disclosures from the Rage Action Group).

Patients undergoing lumpectomy or mastectomy don't usually have to stay in hospital long – a few days, if that, in the case of lumpectomy; a week, or sometimes less, for mastectomy. In the best centres, they will routinely be offered counselling during this period (or better still, before the operation) and are likely to meet the radiation oncologist shortly after discharge from hospital, if they have not already done so. Before radiotherapy starts, the patient's treatment has to be planned with particular care, since all breasts are different and the anatomy of the surrounding area is complex, with many sensitive structures nearby.

Patients will usually attend just one planning session, at which all the measurements are taken, and often an outline of their breast as well, in order that the measurements, physics, calculations and necessary computing for definition of the best possible radiation field arrangement can be completed quickly, with the treatment itself commencing just a few days later. Generally, but not always, patients are recommended to have daily treatment, five days a week, for three to six weeks, depending on the local preferences in the centre they are attending. The treatment volume will always include the whole of the breast, but when a full axillary lymph node dissection has been performed surgically, there is no need to irradiate the axilla (armpit area) at all; in fact, there are good reasons to stay away from it, since long-term lymphoedema (swelling of the arm, from excess tissue fluid) is likely to result from over-treatment of this area.

SIDE-EFFECTS

In the short term, patients can expect to remain pretty well throughout the treatment, though most will experience a slight reddening and/or discomfort in the treated area. For some patients, the skin colour change is more pronounced, more particularly in the pale skinned, and the outermost layer of skin may even partially peel off (dry desquamation), though more serious skin damage (moist desquamation) should not occur to any great extent, except in patients with large, pendulous breasts, where it may be difficult to avoid because of the apposition of skin surfaces at the under-surface of the breast. It can also occur in the axilla, where the dose is high. In any event, these changes should be pretty short lived. The other treatment complications are minor but worth mentioning – many patients feel tired and need to be reassured that this is normal, particularly in the latter half of treatment. Some may feel nauseated, particularly at the start of treatment, though this settles down rapidly and is not generally a problem.

In my view, patients who wish to continue working should be strongly encouraged to do so, since this helps many to sustain their sense of self-esteem, and avoids too much undesirable focusing on the illness at a time when the goal must surely be to get on and complete the course of radiotherapy with as little upset and interruption as possible. The alternative to continuing with work is often an undesirable loss of self-confidence, and all too frequently one sees a disconsolate patient who feels that they are doing the right thing by 'resting', but becomes bored, irritable and anxious. It all depends on the individual, of course – some welcome an opportunity to take time off, particularly where the work is stressful and cannot easily be performed in a half-hearted way. The ideal, I think, is for patients to continue working for, say, the morning and then leave early, coming into the department for treatment on the way home. I think this kind of detail is important, since it helps patients to retain a sense of control over their own lives, a key feature, it seems to me, of successfully coming to terms with a dangerous and unpredictable illness which, perhaps only a month or two beforehand, had not, in all probability, been discovered.

Many patients undergoing radiotherapy will be advised not to wash the affected area. This advice should be taken seriously, since many radiotherapists (myself among them) believe that skin reactions can sometimes be worse in patients who continue to wash, possibly due to the friction and force of towel drying rather than to any more abstruse theoretical reason (though there are theoretical reasons, as well, for believing that skin should be kept dry during treatment). In good departments, patients will be seen and reviewed by one of the medical team on a regular weekly basis (more often, if necessary) so that important details such as skin reaction can be discussed and, if necessary, treated – generally with low-strength hydrocortisone cream, which usually works very well. Most skin reactions settle very quickly, and, after completion of the radiotherapy, patients should expect to be called back to the clinic every three months or so for further review and, in particular, clinical examination. Opinions are divided as to whether further routine mammogram tests should be undertaken during this period, but there is an increasing feeling that it is sensible to repeat them every eighteen to twenty-four months, largely to keep a close watch on the other breast as well as checking the previously irradiated one. It is certainly helpful to have a post-treatment baseline mammogram (at about three to six months) to compare with future views.

OTHER TYPES OF TREATMENT

Before turning to other types of treatment, I should point out that there is more and more evidence that the initial staging procedures in patients with breast cancer can quite reasonably be kept very limited. There was certainly a vogue for performing a whole series of investigations, including abdominal ultrasound examination, isotope bone scanning and a wide variety of blood tests in all cases; we now know that the pick-up rate of these tests is so low that the cost cannot be justified – indeed, some patients suffer considerable anxiety, since the tests can give a 'false positive' picture. Although breast cancer cells can, of course, spread at a microscopic level extremely widely, both to the axillary (and neck) lymph nodes and, even more important, via the bloodstream to distant parts of the body (bone, liver, lung, brain and so on), these potential sites cannot usually be recognised by our current scanning or blood-testing techniques, again arguing in favour of avoiding the tests altogether. We urgently need a better way of establishing whether patients do have secondary spread; a reliable tumour marker would obviously be best, but at the moment no such substance has emerged. The best guide to future events is the presence and degree of lymph node involvement of the axilla, with a strong body of evidence that it is capable of providing a quantitative estimate of the outcome. Patients with ten positive lymph nodes clearly do worse, as a group, than those with five nodes, who in turn have a less satisfactory prognosis than those with only one or two positive nodes.

Apart from the revolution in local treatment which has led so rapidly to rejection of mastectomy as the 'gold standard', an equally dramatic series of developments has led to the majority of patients now being treated with prophylactic or adjuvant systemic therapy – drug treatment, either with chemotherapy, hormone therapy or both – in an attempt to forestall the development of life-threatening metastases. As mentioned earlier, many patients with breast cancer harbour micro-metastases, microscopic deposits which cannot be visualised, but are present at the outset of the disease and not, of course, amenable to any form of local therapy, be it surgery or radiation.

It became clear almost ten years ago that the routine use of tamoxifen, a simple tablet preparation taken daily for two years or more, could protect post-menopausal breast cancer patients (i.e. seventy-five per cent of all cases), not to anything like a complete degree but sufficient to justify this treatment as an essential part of management in post-menopausal women. Tamoxifen is a well-tolerated oral agent, developed in the UK and now used world-wide, which was initially thought to act solely through its anti-oestrogenic properties, i.e. by depriving any residual breast cancer cells of the essential oestrogen which they required for continued growth. It now seems likely that tamoxifen does more than this, since patients who have oestrogen receptor negative tumours (i.e. with no evidence of a hormonal dependence, using a simple test now widely available) do sometimes still respond, though admittedly less frequently than oestrogen receptor positive patients.

Over the past few years, evidence has been mounting that tamoxifen is probably also valuable in the pre-menopausal patient as well, and many of us (myself included) use it routinely for all patients with breast cancer, regardless of age. Some would argue that patients with a particularly good prognosis (small primary tumour, no lymph node involvement despite a full axillary node dissection) do so well that tamoxifen is not justifiable in this group. I would certainly not argue with this if the patient in question is pre-menopausal, though my personal view is that, for post-menopausal patients, the benefits of tamoxifen are so clear that no patient should be denied the potential benefit unless they are among the very small group who find tamoxifen impossible to cope with.

Side-effects are very few, but include weight gain, occasional nausea, vaginal bleeding or discharge (usually very mild, but sometimes worrying for the patient – both of these symptoms generally settle down), and symptoms resulting from the oestrogen blockade, such as changes to the hair, skin or nails. Tamoxifen is not a contraceptive, and patients are likely to remain potentially fertile, even though in some brands of the drugs, the package insert claims that periods do stop. In my experience, they generally don't, though there may be a real benefit for patients who, for much of their lives, may have suffered from irregular periods, as they often discover that, with tamoxifen, their periods are more or less normal – a real bonus. Other, much rarer side-effects include reduction in the platelet count (thrombocytopenia – discussed more fully in chapter 20) and a sudden and potentially serious elevation in the circulating calcium level (hypercalcaemia), which I have only seen once or twice, despite having prescribed tamoxifen literally thousands of times. In the long term, there is certainly a very small risk of tamoxifen-related increase in the incidence of uterine cancer, presumably because tamoxifen's complex action includes some pro-oestrogenic as well as anti-oestrogenic effects (so much so that tamoxifen is sometimes used in infertility clinics!); again, this side-effect is extremely unusual and, in my view, does not begin to compare as a potential disadvantage with the life-saving properties of the drug in patients with breast cancer.

One important and still unanswered question is just how long the tamoxifen should be given for. The very important Cancer Research Campaign study currently running for post-menopausal patients is addressing the two- versus five-year question, though some specialists feel that tamoxifen is so beneficial that it should be given indefinitely. I do not personally subscribe to this view, since I simply don't believe we have the necessary information; and if there really is a risk from the point of view of uterine cancer, it could multiply to a much more significant level in patients who are taking tamoxifen for many years. The two- versus five-year question seems to me to be the right one, though I must declare an interest here, since I am a member of the Cancer Research Campaign breast cancer trials committee. I should also point out that there are alternative forms of adjuvant hormone therapy, notably the use of a radiation or surgically induced menopause, which again has a solid weight of evidence to support it. Most specialists (and patients) feel, however, that tamoxifen is simpler and more generally acceptable.

The other major type of systemic adjuvant therapy is, of course, chemotherapy, which has attracted so much attention in the past few years. Like tamoxifen, it has now been used for about two decades, but only recently taken up enthusiastically in the UK, by an essentially conservative profession. The original view was that such treatment was simply too toxic to be taken seriously, but again, the weight of evidence is now very strongly in favour of chemotherapy as standard adjuvant treatment for all pre-menopausal patients with lymph node positive disease. In this group, chemotherapy can be shown to improve survival, though patients with only one or two positive lymph nodes do almost as well as those with negative nodes, and some specialists would regard the use of chemotherapy in this group as being too intensive, though I do not myself agree. Apart from the unequivocal increase in survival in lymph node positive, pre-menopausal patients, there is also evidence that, even in the node negative group (who do much better anyway), there is an increase in what is termed 'disease-free survival', i.e. the probability of a patient remaining clear of recurrent disease, either at the original site or elsewhere, during the follow-up period. It may seem self-evident that any lengthening of disease-free survival should automatically translate into an improvement in the more important, life-or-death, overall survival figure, but in fact this is still far from clear – because of the relative effectiveness of some of the available treatments for patients with recurrent disease. It's an important point because on the one hand, there is a natural tendency to use chemotherapy (or any other potentially useful treatment) for *all* patients who might reasonably bene- fit, but on the other, would it be right and proper to give intensive treatment of this kind to patients who may remain free of disease a little longer, but in whom, ultimately, the overall survival figures can't be shown to be unequivocally better? Life would be much easier, of course, if the treatment were both straightforward, inexpensive and very easy to tolerate and although tamoxifen more or less satisfies these criteria, I don't think the same claim could be made for chemotherapy.

Most pre-menopausal patients under the age of fifty and with node positive disease are now routinely offered chemotherapy, usually with six courses of a standard drug regimen known as CMF (cyclophosphamide, methotrexate, flourouracil), which has been in common use for about twenty years now and was initially pioneered by Italian and American oncologists. With modern anti-nausea drugs, this chemotherapy is generally very well tolerated, almost invariably given on an out-patient basis and at approximately three- to four-week intervals, i.e. over a period of just under six months, provided that the blood count remains satisfactory throughout. Side-effects are described in chapter 5 (page 57).

Although CMF is very well researched and its effects understood in considerable depth, we're constantly on the lookout for superior treatments which might yield better results, paticularly in the higher risk groups such as patients with a very large number of positive axillary lymph nodes in the operative specimen. More powerful agents might well be recommended right from the start, possibly as part of a clinical trial. It might be, for example, that the researchers are interested in a possible advantage in giving the drugs on a continuous, infusional basis – through a Hickman line, perhaps – rather than the traditional, intermittent pulse approach with chemotherapy. At present, though, despite encouraging reports from the USA and elsewhere, it is far from proven that more intensive chemotherapy than CMF has definite superiority, at least in the majority of patients without adverse risk features such as major axillary node involvement. One much-heralded approach is the use of very high-dose chemotherapy supplemented by autologous bone marrow transplantation or peripheral stem cell transfusion (see chapter 5) for high-risk breast cancer patients, a treatment pioneered by Professor Bill Peters in North Carolina (USA) and now more widely available on the NHS in this country. Although the initial results are extremely encouraging, the only comparison so far is with 'historical controls' rather than with a contemporary randomised group of patients treated by the best current conventional chemotherapy. Until these results are available, it would be unwise ro regard the exciting new high-dose techniques as the treatment of choice. Randomised trials will provide the most reliable answer!

Some patients, probably the majority, will find that their menstrual cycle is substantially disrupted by chemotherapy, often to the point of complete cessation of periods. The closer the patient is to her expected menopause, the more likely this is to occur. Younger women given chemotherapy should be warned that it does not act as a contraceptive, nor is it likely to completely abolish the periods, even though they might be disrupted during the treatment itself. In young women, fertility is likely to be preserved, and there are many instances of patients becoming pregnant afterwards. The question of whether or not the induction of a 'chemical' menopause of this kind is truly beneficial remains one of the uncertainties in this whole area. Soem specialists believe that chemotherapy chiefly works via its effect on the ovary, so that if the patient continues to menstruate after six months' chemotherapy, the treatment should be augmented by pelvic irradiation or surgical removal of the ovaries, to be on the safe side, so to speak. I don't myself share this view, but it is quite widely held, particularly abroad.

The trouble with the induction of the menopause at an early age is that it can produce sudden and very undesirable symptomatic side-effects – troublesome and persistent hot flushes, loss of libido, a tendency towards earlier osteoporosis and a group of symptoms related to chronological ageing which some patients find hard to cope with. But to some extent, these can be prevented by the use of low-dose progesterone administration, such as Provera 20 milligrams daily, which seems to work well with the majority of patients, (though not all) and which, as far as one can tell, is completely safe. There is even an increasing view, quite contrary to traditional teaching, that Hormone Replacement Therapy (HRT) is not unreasonable in selected patients who are greatly upset by the onset of this menopause. It may seem illogical to first produce a menopause deliberately and then offer hormone replacement but in truth, there may be some sense to it, since, for example, symptomatic HRT benefits can occur even though the dose of HRT, given in tablet or patch form, is substantially lower than the level of circulating oestrogens which have been medically lowered. Once again, views on this difficult issue are divided, and there are certainly no worthwhile trials of the use of HRT in patients with breast cancer which would guide us to a firm conclusion. My own practice, and that of many of my colleagues, would be to avoid routine HRT wherever possible, but to use either progesterones or conventional HRT in selected symptomatic patients who requested it, or for patients in whom there is a strong family history of osteoporosis which could represent a real threat to their future health. There is no doubt that the quality of life is in many respects much imporved by the administration of HRT, a key issue in the decision-making process.

TREATMENT FOR RECURRENT DISEASE

Sadly, many patients with breast cancer do develop a recurrent disease, either at the primary site (though this is much less common these days) or as a result of distant spread, for example in the bones of the spine, ribs, pelvis or femur (thigh bone), or the lung, skin or brain. Obviously, the clinical features will vary widely, depending on the precise site and degree of involvement; it is impossible to list here the ways in which such secondary spread might become apparent, though these are discussed to some extent in chapter 3. As far as treatment of secondary recurrence is concerned, the important thing, of course, is to weigh up the pros and cons of additional treatment with great care, and use only those methods which are likely to be symptomatically beneficial for the patient. For the most part, and certainly in the case of distant secondary spread, cure is unfortunately no longer possible. It is, however, quite surprising how often the rule of 'first do no harm' is ignored, sometimes by enthusiasts (not always oncologists) who may have and inflative view of what palliative chemotherapy might be able to achieve. Although there is a natural tendency to recommend treatment in every case, one needs to keep a clear head as to what, realistically, might be the consequences – both beneficial and harmful. For instance, in a patient with a severe and focal (localised) discomfort as a result of a secondary deposit in a rib, a single dose of radiotherapy to the painful site will often produce excellent pain relief with little, if anything, in the way of troublesome side-effects. In general, radiotherapy offers and excellent chance of local pain control with bone secondaries at any site. A surgical stabilisation (internal orthopaedic fixation of a long bone, such as the femur for example) may also be useful in conjunction with radiotherapy. On the other hand, radiotherapy is difficult to use for abdominal secondary deposits, such as those arising within the liver, because of the limited tolerance of this organ and the close proximity of other very sensitive structures. In these circumstances, chemotherapy is more likely to be valuable, even in patients who have received previous adjuvant chemotherapy. If radiotherapy is the cornerstone of the treatment for bone and brain secondaries, chemotherapy (or possibly a change of hormone therapy, especially in patients known to be hormone responsive) is, on the whole, a better choice for lung, liver and/or glandular secondary deposits.

Patients with advanced or recurrent breast cancer also quite often respond to alterations in their hormonal medication, and there is a wide variety of agents available. Most patients will have had treatment with tamoxifen as part of the initial or primary management; whilst some will have discontinued this treatment at the time of their relapse, others develop evidence of progressive disease whilst still taking it. For the first of these groups, particularly where they have been off the tamoxifen for several years beforehand, it makes excellent sense to restart treatment with tamoxifen, since there may be an additional response. If, on the other hand, the relapse has occurred whilst the patient is actually taking it, there is little point in continuing with it, or at least relying on it as the sole treatment. In these circumstances, the advice is usually to switch to a second-line hormone such as progesterone (typically given in much higher dosage that that used for symptomatic treatment of hot flushes) or an agent called aminoglutethimide, which prevents the normal mechanism of steroid manufacture in the adrenal glands, thus reducing the sex steroid synthesis as well. This needs to be supplemented by cortisone, since it also blocks the production of cortisone from the adrenal, and for this reason is a slightly more complicated agent to use. Although all of these drugs can be given by mouth, there are one or two other choices which are typically given by fortnightly or monthly injections.

BREAST CANCER PROGNOSIS

Much has been written about the outlook or prognosis in breast cancer patients. Certainly it is one of the more unpredictable tumours, in the sense that patients who are free of disease, apparently cured, at five years after treatment, are not quite in the smae position as those with, say, lung or testis cancer; after five years free of these cancers, patients are almost certainly genuinely out of the woods. With breast cancer, it's rather different, since the disease can return at a later stage. This may be tough and unwelcome news, but although breast cancer is unusual in this regard, *most* of the relapses which occur, do so within the first five years – some comfort, at least. It's also true that, on the whole, the later the disease recurs, the more likely the patient is to respond effectively to additional treatment when required – as if the tempo of the disease has a considerable bearing, not only on its virulence, but also on the final outcome. It was the recognition that breast cancer can return many years later, at a distant site from the initial tumour, that led so many experts to begin to question the key importance of mastectomy in the first place. It took far too many decades, and far too many unnecessary operations, for the medical profession to recognise that the real problem in breast cancer was not so much related to the difficulty in local control in the first place, but rather the late, distant recurrence which might prove fatal. Certainly in terms of prognosis, the smaller the tumour the more likely the patient is to be cured by the initial choice of treatment. Other important determinants are the lymph node status (whether positive or negative) as determined by the surgical dissection of the axillary nodes (generally regarded as the most important prognostic feature of all) and the pathological 'grade' of the tumour, i.e. the degree of visible abnormalities in the cancer cells when viewed under the microscope. Some look very similar to normal breast tissue, others very bizarre.

The huge world-wide epidemic of breast cancer, so marked in the industrialised Western nations, has led to an explosion of research work. Although many are gloomy about the slow rate of change, the past fifteen years or so have seen at least two major advances with real benefits for the majority of patients: the recognition that mastectomy is often quite unnecessary and can be replaced by a much simpler and less destructive operation; and secondly, the recognition that systemic agents such as tamoxifen and chemotherapy are clearly capable of reducing the recurrence and death rates. It's hard to predict what the next decade may bring, but certainly there are reasons, in my view, to be cautiously optimistic about future progress.

Case histories

ELIZABETH'S STORY

Like many women, Elizabeth was well aware of the high prevalence of breast cancer and examined her breasts every month. A married teacher with three daughters and now in charge of the Maths Department at a large London school, she was extremely anxious about a lump she thought she detected after getting out of her bath one morning. Like her husband, Elizabeth's doctor was unconvinced and not terribly keen to refer her to a breast clinic.

However, she insisted, and an examination by the specialist, together with a mammogram, revealed a 2-centimetre mass which clearly had to come out. First, though, she had to cope with the terrible wait following the fine needle aspiration (it would have to be a Bank Holiday!) and, worse, the news that the fine needle test had proven 'suspicious but not conclusive'. There was nothing for it – the test had to be repeated; unless, of course, she would like to have the lump surgically removed, which might well be necessary anyway. But she wasn't very keen to have this done – in the first place, she didn't want a permanent 3-centimetre scar if it wasn't strictly necessary, and secondly, her breasts were on the small side, and she didn't want bits removed unless they really had to come out. Further delay followed (and a terrible night with a duodenal ulcer which she thought she'd seen the last of) before she finally received the positive result she'd been dreading.

Afterwards, she said that the staff couldn't have been kinder, but she knew at the time she was going to pieces. Because of the size of her breasts, the surgeon recommended a mastectomy, although wide local excision of the cancer, with preservation of the breast and post-operative radiotherapy might be possible. But educated, informed and supported as she was, Elizabeth felt quite unable to make such a weighty decision for herself. It was simply more than she could cope with. She wasn't at all sure she could deal with the loss of her breast, and yet it might be the only way of saving her life. Would the promised breast reconstruction really restore her previous figure, or was she, at forty-two, doomed to an impossibly rapid physical decline? And would her husband, who only two years previously had left her for six months claiming he needed 'more personal space' and then unexpectedly returned, stay for good this time?

She accepted the mastectomy, the reconstruction and the post-operative treatment with good grace but a heavy heart. Three (out of twenty) of the axillary lymph nodes had contained secondary tumours, so chemotherapy, which she had been warned might be necessary, was clearly indicated in order to reduce her risk of recurrence and improve her prospects for overall survival. Somewhat unexpectedly, she found the chemotherapy – normally a pretty straightforward affair and given on an out-patient basis – extremely tough. It did help to have the treatment on a Friday so she could use the weekend to get over it before school started again on Monday, but despite our reassurances and confident predictions, she felt well below par about fifty per cent of the time during that six-month period, far more than the three or four days per month we had outlined. 'But it's a good way of losing weight,' she told us.

She bounced back without too much trouble, and the first three years of follow-up went extremely well, though sadly and much to her embarrassment, her husband did indeed disappear, this time for good, with another man. Three months later, as I called her in for what I'd hoped would be a routine consultation, I noticed that she staggered as she got up from her chair and walked clumsily into my room, knocking her elbow on the door frame. She'd been aware of slight dizziness and poor balance, but had not noticed double vision, headache or weakness. It wasn't easy explaining to her that things weren't right, and that I was suspicious that she might have a secondary deposit within the brain.

The brain scan unfortunately confirmed what I'd guessed at, and showed several sites of secondary cancer, the largest in the cerebellum at the back of the brain, the area responsible for balance and co-ordination. She was devastated. She wept for the first time and told me that she'd not told either her mother or her two younger daughters about her cancer, having sworn her eldest (aged twenty-three and a student teacher herself) to secrecy. 'But they'll have to know now, won't they?' she said.

I agreed. I certainly wasn't sure how much I should tell her at this stage of her prognosis, since she already had so much on her plate, and ideally her daughter, or somebody else close to her, should be there when I broke the news.

Not all stories have a happy ending, and Elizabeth died of progressive cancer six months after we had completed a course of radiotherapy to the whole brain. It caused loss of hair, but happily this had regrown by the time of her death, and the six months she had gained were sufficient for her to tell her mother, daughters and her estranged husband (whom she knew would once again be in charge of the girls) about her illness and her dashed hopes. When she died in the local hospice, all of them were around her bed.

Breast cancer is a strange illness. Unlike Elizabeth, her neighbour Gwen (just six doors down in the same street) seemed very unlikely to do well when we first met.

GWEN'S STORY

Gwen was thirty-seven when I first encountered her, a painter with a lengthy history of profound psychological disturbance and several serious suicide attempts. She was divorced, had no children, was introspective and emotionally unstable. She'd been well aware of a substantial lump in her breast for at least six months before finally going to see her GP, ostensibly with the quite unrelated problem of sleeplessness and daily fatigue. It was only as she was about to leave that she mentioned the lump. It was enormous, occupying almost all of her left breast. Although it hadn't ulcerated yet, it wouldn't have been more than a couple of weeks. The specialist who saw her the following day couldn't feel any glands under the arm and surprisingly, the operation proved straightforward. She declined both radiotherapy and chemotherapy, but agreed to take tamoxifen and to see us regularly for follow-up treatment.

That was seven years ago. Since that time, she has never missed a visit, hasn't looked back and psychologically seems healthier than before. Every couple of years, I get an invitation to her latest exhibition. She obviously enjoys confounding the statistics, but I think she knows as well as I do that, with breast cancer, you can never be quite sure.

It's interesting how many patients like Gwen do seem to find a new focus in their lives when faced with a truly desperate, potentially life-threatening illness.

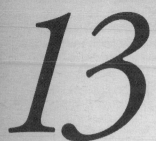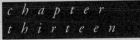

chapter thirteen

BRAIN TUMOURS

B rain tumours are perhaps the most feared of all human cancers. After all, the brain is the seat of the human mind, and is widely understood as the most sophisticated of all our organs. How could the body possibly withstand or recover from such a dreadful illness as a malignancy within the very nerve centre of the human frame?

Causes of brain tumours

Brain tumours affect both children and adults, and vary widely in their type and clinical development. Children's brain tumours are described in chapter 24; for adults, the peak age incidence is fifty to sixty years, and almost nothing is known of the causation or background, apart from the very small group of cerebral (i.e. 'arising from the brain') lymphomas which can occur in patients with profoundly lowered immunity. These are the brain tumours that can arise in patients with AIDS or those in whom long-term suppression of immunity is deliberately produced by medication, for example in patients with an organ transplant, to avoid rejection of the donated organ.

These cases are very unusual compared with the far more common group of 'gliomas', a word which embraces the commoner types of brain tumour. The term glioma means that the cancer has arisen from the nervous tissue of the brain itself or of the supporting structures within the brain. Taken together, these cases account for over ninety per cent of all primary brain tumours (and, for that matter, spinal cord tumours as well, though these are genuinely rare). The characteristic type of tumour in adults is quite different from the childhood types and, overall, a great deal more common.

One curious feature of adult brain tumours is that they rarely spread or disseminate to other parts of the body, a major difference between brain tumours and most other types of cancer which has never been fully explained, though there are plenty of theories. Since spread beyond the initial, or primary, site is generally felt to be a fundamental and defining feature of most types of cancer, brain tumours clearly contravene this general principle. This does not, unfortunately, make them any less malignant, since local control, even by radical surgery and/or radiotherapy, is often extremely difficult to achieve. This is discussed in greater detail in the section on *Treatment*.

Symptoms and diagnosis

Patients with brain tumours can be diagnosed in a variety of ways, and symptoms range from the subtle to the devastating – the site of the cancer will invariably dictate the pattern of symptoms. For example, patients with tumours situated in the highest area, near the vertex of the skull, may have a weakness of the arm or leg, just as if they had had a stroke, since this area of the brain is concerned with motor function, and the tumour will displace this area quite markedly, particularly if there is a substantial local reaction around the tumour, as is often the case. Because of 'cross-over' of the major nervous pathways from brain to spinal cord, tumours situated in the right half of the brain (the right hemisphere) produce left-sided weakness or sensory loss, and vice versa. Even small tumours can produce quite devastating neurological symptoms if situated in the appropriate area, in marked contrast to others, where a less critically important area of the brain is affected. These areas are sometimes referred to as 'silent' areas of the brain, and a good example is the frontal lobe, long known to be the main representational area for personality, intellect and self-control, but with a less clear-cut role with regard to touch, sensation, muscular power or sight. Tumours situated at the back of the brain, in the cerebellum or brain stem (situated more or less at the junction of the brain and spine, and containing much of the most complicated nervous circuitry passing down from the brain to the varying levels of spinal cord) often produce symptoms of poor balance or other complicated neurological syndromes.

Brain tumours can grow quite slowly, particularly those of low pathological grade, i.e. tumours where the appearance under the microscope shows very little departure from the normal pattern of brain tissue. In other cases, particularly for the most malignant types known as 'glioblastoma multiforme', the microscopic appearance, by contrast, shows a much more disordered and bizarre cellular arrangement, quite unlike normal brain tissue, and with a much more elaborate blood supply. It is generally not too difficult for a pathologist to describe the tumour grade, and most hospitals use a grading system dividing primary brain tumours into four types, from the least to the most malignant. The symptomatic history is likely to be much shorter with tumours of higher grade (3 or 4) but with grade 1 or grade 2 tumours, the patient may have suffered a very slowly evolving clinical history, often over many years, typically suffering also from epilepsy if the tumour is situated in the appropriate part of the brain.

I am not suggesting that every patient with epilepsy has a brain tumour – far from it. It is, however, important for epileptics to have a brain scan at some point, since a small but critically sited brain tumour may be responsible for the symptoms, and it is always worth making sure. As with so many types of cancer, it is far easier to deal with a small tumour than a big one; indeed, it may even make all the difference between cure and failure. Some types of tumour, notably those situated in the temporal lobe or underside part of the brain, can cause curious hallucinatory types of epilepsy, in which the patient might, for example, have a very strong sense of a smell which nobody else can detect, or a foreboding of some terrible impending disaster. I remember one patient with a temporal lobe tumour who had overwhelming hallucinations affecting her sense of smell. Unfortunately the smell she experienced was of fire and smoke, and she had raised the alarm and emptied the building where she worked (a large comprehensive school) on five separate occasions before one of the teachers realised something was up.

Others of my patients have likened the olfactory hallucination (i.e. delusional sense of smell) to strawberries, peppers, acid or, in one odd case (in a wine buff), a 1969 Burgundy. It's all in the brain somewhere! Some patients with a brain tumour continually bump into things, from a loss of part of the visual field as a result of the tumour interrupting the visual pathways within the brain. Since these are unusually lengthy, from the eye to the computing area for sight situated very far back in the occipital lobe, there is plenty of opportunity for this to happen. I have known cases where the first symptom of the brain tumour was that the patient, normally a careful and courteous driver, repeatedly drove into the kerb or onto the pavement because he was simply unable to comprehend that a consistent part of his visual field had been lost.

The other important groups of brain tumour symptoms are those relating to pressure. It is often not appreciated that the skull is a remarkably rigid structure which encloses the brain completely. For this reason, any area within the brain which expands – not only from a tumour; it can just as easily be a sudden haemorrhage or clot – will, as a result, produce an increase in the 'intracranial' pressure, since there is simply nowhere for the extra volume to be accommodated. It is for this reason that patients with brain tumours so frequently complain of headaches; other important pressure-related symptoms include nausea, vomiting and double vision. Neurologists and other specialists often look for increased intracranial pressure by careful inspection of the back of the eye, since the optic nerve – the nerve from the brain to the retina – is able to transmit excess pressure, with a characteristic appearance ('papilloe-dema') of the optic disc, which will permit rapid diagnosis of this raised pressure. Once again, it is the site of the tumour, rather than its precise size or nature, which is likely to determine whether or not these symptoms are present.

The fluid part of the brain (the ventricles) are in direct communication with the spinal canal and the spinal cord, and any interruption or blockage is likely to lead to increased fluid pressure (internal hydro-cephalus) and early pressure symptoms. Even a small tumour, if situated in the appropriate area near the outflow point of the ventricles, is likely to do this, whereas quite large tumours, if situated in the outer or more solid part of the brain may not produce these symptoms at all.

Not all brain tumours are malignant. For example, tumours of the pituitary gland, arising from the hormonally active gland ('the size of a Heinz baked bean', as one of my chiefs used to say) at the bottom of the brain, are always benign. They nonetheless belong to a very important group, since they can produce terrible symptoms, either by hormone under- or over-production or by simple expansion leading to dangerous pressure on surrounding structures. Sitting just above and in front of the gland, for example, is one of the most important parts of the nervous network between eye and brain, the optic chiasm, and interruption of this structure can lead to permanent loss of vision, usually resulting in a very characteristic visual field alteration, known as a 'hemianopia' because half of the visual field will be lost, and the other half perfectly retained. This is the type of patient who bumps into things or, unaware of the defect, drives into a kerb or lamppost. Other types of benign brain tumour include those on the covering layers of the brain, the meninges; a so-called meningoma is often one of the more gratifying brain tumours to treat, since it is often possible to shell these out very successfully by skilled neurosurgery.

The diagnosis of brain tumours has undergone a revolution over the past twenty years, with the advent of CT and then MRI scanning (see chapter 4). Before these techniques became available, it was often necessary to rely entirely on clinical judgement, always a dangerous policy, or to use investigational techniques which were often painful and could be dangerous. Nowadays, with modern scanning techniques, we are able to gain remarkably detailed pictures of most brain tumours, and with the added advantage that these investigations can be repeated if necessary, for example after treatment has been completed, in order to assess what has been achieved.

Apart from the technical quality and, dare I say it, the aesthetic beauty of the scans, their real value lies in the enormous advantage they give the brain surgeon or specialist radiotherapist who naturally wish to deal with the tumour as effectively as possible, but without disrupting local surrounding structures any more than is strictly necessary. Many more tumours can now, at least, be biopsied more safely than before, giving much needed information on the type of tumour, even though it may not be possible to go further and remove it entirely. This may involve using a special stereotactic frame, attached to the patient's head, to allow needle biopsy (under scanning control) of a tumour which is not amenable to any other type of surgery. This particularly applies to those in the 'dominant' hemisphere of the brain, i.e. the side which contains the speech area, generally the left-hand side of the brain. Most surgeons would be much more prepared to remove tumours on the right ('non-dominant') side than the left, for fear of causing permanent damage without real benefit to offset the drawbacks. Unfortunately, brain tumours are as common in the dominant as in the non-dominant hemisphere.

Treatment

Although diagnosis of brain tumours has become more and more straightforward with the wide availability of CT and MRI scanning, the same cannot be said of treatment. There remains a wide variety of views among neurologists, neurosurgeons and oncological specialists, some taking the view that treatment results are too poor to justify routine intervention, with all the attendant dangers, whereas others adopt a much more positive approach, following the philosophy that the negative or nihilistic view will inevitably result, sooner or later, in failure to treat a tumour that could have been cured. With low-grade tumours, for example, the outlook is not too bad, at least for an elderly person, since many patients will survive for years or even decades following initial treatment with either surgery or radiotherapy (or sometimes both). On the other hand, those less convinced of the benefits of immediate treatment point to the patients with low-grade brain tumours whom they have followed over several years, using repeat CT scanning, but without active intervention unless the tumour enlarges or the symptoms become severe.

Although the matter has never been formally settled by a proper comparative study, my own view is that most of these patients do benefit from early treatment, and I have certainly seen many cases of low-grade brain tumour in which the patient has struggled for years with recurrent epilepsy symptoms, often very difficult to control, but rapidly improved by radiotherapy, even if the tumour was too large or too dangerously situated to attempt surgical resection. It is therefore possible, in my view, to justify treatment on symptomatic grounds, even if an improvement in overall survival cannot be guaranteed. The drawback for radiotherapy in such patients is the inevitable hair loss which is caused by the X-ray beam passing through the scalp; the higher the dose, the slower the regrowth. Psychologically, however, it seems to me that more and more patients are preferring the active approach, understandably (to my mind) declaring themselves dissatisfied with the prospect of simply living with the tumour for an indefinite period, and undergoing treatment at a later stage, only when the symptoms become intolerable. The difficulty, of course, is that brain tumours, whether low or high grade, are generally not among the more responsive of tumours to radiotherapy (but with some important exceptions, particularly in the childhood group – see chapter 24), so the benefits are likely to be limited.

The same general points apply, perhaps with even greater force, to high-grade brain tumours, where the prognosis is regrettably so much poorer, even if active treatment is carried out. Patients with these tumours really do have the cards stacked against them, particularly with the very high grade (glioblastoma multiforme) cases, where cure is almost unknown. But this does not, in my view, mean that nothing can or should be attempted. First of all, patients with high-grade brain tumours need time, both for themselves and their families, to adjust to this devastating and probably fatal condition; such time can only be offered if the specialist treating the patient can at least recommend or point to a coherent treatment policy. It may be that the patient only has a few months to live, but what important months they are. Secondly, the quality of life is, in my judgement, likely to be improved by treatment.

I realise, of course, that the time spent in hospital following a major brain operation may well interfere with this, and the same applies in principle for radiotherapy attendances; on the other hand, however, the quality of a life in which the patient knows full well that he or she is simply waiting, often unaided, for the end seems to me grossly impaired as well. Active treatment does at least allow for a positive and pugnacious approach which most patients, their partners and families find rewarding at the time, even if ultimately a failure. And then thirdly, you get the odd surprise. I remember, for example, a high-flying barrister, struck down by a very high-grade brain tumour, who found it difficult to decide whether or not to agree to active treatment. In the event, he decided to go for it, and lived for another fifteen months, much of the time spent on his feet in the courtroom, winning a couple of cases that he had almost given up on, and with the large bald area from the radiotherapy very adequately covered by his barrister's wig. In cases such as these, it is often the family who benefit as greatly as the patient. There is nothing so depressing as feeling guiltily (rightly or wrongly) after the death of a loved one that important approaches might have been left unexplored.

In some cases, chemotherapy will be recommended by the specialist. The present position is that, whilst both surgery and radiotherapy are generally accepted forms of treatment for brain tumours, chemotherapy has a much more uncertain role. There are no drugs currently available which have a really profound effect on the tumour, but those which we have do appear, from time to time, to exert a benefit. In the UK, the Medical Research Council (the MRC) is running an excellent study in which patients are being randomised to receive chemotherapy (in addition to surgery and radiotherapy) in an attempt to see whether or not these patients really do benefit. I strongly support this, since there is clearly no other way to settle the question (and the whole issue is more fully discussed in chapter 6). The chemotherapy that we use does occasionally cause nausea and vomiting, but the side-effects are, in general, not too troublesome, and we certainly need to know the answer.

The other drug which is very widely used in brain tumours is dexamethasone. This is the most potent steroid we have, and, like all steroids, is a potentially dangerous agent. However, its results with brain tumours are often miraculous, and I have known many patients whose lives have been transformed. It acts by reducing the local swelling ('cerebral oedema'), rapidly relieving symptoms of raised intracranial pressure and often improving the patient out of all recognition. The trouble is that these early benefits of dexamethasone turn into disadvantages if the drug is given for too long, since we then see all the steroid side-effects, such as muscle weakness, weight gain, fluid retention, easy bruising and so on. Fortunately, it is usually possible to gradually reduce the steroid dose during the post-operative period, and even sometimes during the three- to six-week course of radiotherapy, so that it can be tailed off completely, generally within six weeks or so after completion of the radiotherapy, without the terrible symptoms returning. If patients relapse at a later stage, at a time when further radiotherapy or surgery cannot be attempted, dexamethasone is likely to be the most valuable drug for palliation of the patient's symptoms, even though life expectancy will probably be very short.

The brain is a relatively common site for secondary deposits of cancer. The important difference, of course, is that in these cases, the primary tumour has arisen elsewhere, for example in the breast or lung, and the tumour may have spread to various other sites as well. These secondary tumours are quite different in their fundamental characteristics from the primary brain tumours outlined in this chapter, and, if biopsied, show just the same characteristics of the original tumour from breast, lung or wherever, rather than the quite different appearances of a primary tumour arising from the brain itself. They are often multiple, rather than the typically single abnormality seen with primary brain tumours and are treated rather differently. First of all, neurosurgical removal is rarely worth considering, though there are some important exceptions, notably patients where there is a single secondary deposit, and, best of all, where extensive investigations show no other evidence of disease at any additional site, particularly if a lengthy interval has elapsed between the original diagnosis and the appearance of the secondary deposit in the brain. Sadly, this only applies in a very small minority of cases, and, for the most part, the treatment decision lies between whole brain irradiation (which can be supported by the use of dexamethasone as outlined earlier) or supportive care with steroids alone, but without the radiotherapy.

Radiotherapy can be very valuable, particularly with tumours that are likely to be rapidly responsive, such as secondary deposits from small cell lung cancer (see chapter 11). On the other hand, the patient will have to accept some degree of hair loss, though not generally long term since the usual convention, quite properly, is to regard treatment of this kind as essentially palliative, without any real prospect of a lasting cure, and therefore best given in a limited dose so as to avoid treatment complications. In some cases, chemotherapy is worth considering as well.

There is no denying that brain tumours do indeed produce devastating symptoms. Hospice and community support teams regard them as being among the most difficult of tumours to deal with, and patients do naturally fear for their sanity as well as their lives. It is never easy to answer the frequently posed question, 'What's going to happen at the end?', but the truth is that many patients drift gradually into an increasingly comatose state, often with little in the way of additional symptoms. A caring general practitioner (if the patient is at home) or other specialist can achieve remarkable quality of care by careful use of dexamethasone, anticonvulsants and other medications; at the very end, it is sometimes kindest to withdraw the steroid therapy and permit the increasing pressure within the brain to deepen the patient's coma still further.

As far as cure is concerned, there is no use pretending that brain tumours are truly curable – in the commonly accepted sense of the word – all that often. But we do have our successes, even with patients with high-grade tumours, of whom a small proportion can undoubtedly be cured, without evidence of further relapse following the initial treatment with surgery and radiotherapy. They may constitute only ten per cent or so of the total group, but how terrible to miss the opportunity even with a single case.

Current research efforts are directed towards the increasing use of neurosurgical imaging and resection, the investigation of chemotherapy (including novel agents only just introduced into clinical practice), and the development of new drugs which might have greater potency. There may be a long way to go, but at least the battle is joined.

Case history

DOMINIC'S STORY

Dominic, aged forty-seven, is second-in-command of a large public company, divorced and remarried, with two young children. Five years ago, he developed a severe headache, blurred vision and nausea, which, he insisted, were work related. He didn't see his GP until three months later, when pressures of work allowed; the GP immediately sought a neurological opinion from a specialist. A week later, a CT brain scan confirmed a large frontal brain tumour, which was removed by a neurosurgeon and turned out to be a low-grade glioma. He made a remarkable recovery and was back on his feet within weeks, once again undertaking weighty decisions, his business skills apparently undiminished.

Four years later, the symptoms returned. Again, he ignored them for six weeks, but his wife insisted that he see the specialist again and was furious to discover that, unbeknown to her, he had discontinued his previous follow-up visits, again due to pressure of work. A new brain scan showed obvious reactivation of the tumour, though the scan from the previous year (at his last follow-up visit) had been normal. This time, the tumour proved unresectable, and a biopsy showed evidence of progression to a higher grade, with a much more serious outlook.

The recommended treatment was a combination of radical radiotherapy and chemotherapy, and Dominic willingly participated in a clinical trial in which the chemotherapy was prospectively randomised (see chapter 6). Once again, he's back at work, now into his sixth cycle of chemotherapy, given on an out-patient basis. Recent brain scans have shown shrinkage of the tumour following his course of radiotherapy, but Dominic and his wife both realise that the disease could still be partly active, even though he has no symptoms.

The disease highlighted several problems within their marriage, but they now seem closer than before; she has overcome her anger at his laid-back attitude, which she felt was partly responsible for the recurrence not being picked up earlier. Although I don't personally feel that much was lost by his shoulder-shrugging attitude, doctors are so fond of saying that early diagnosis is the key, that it's difficult to remain reassuring on this point without sounding totally inconsistent. Although the chemotherapy is well tolerated, Dominic depends more on his wife than before, even for such simple things as getting to and from the hospital, so she now has more of a role in his life than previously, which she certainly appreciates. Having spent far more time at home as result of the illness than he ever did before, Dominic also realises – a bit grudgingly, perhaps – that running the home isn't quite the plain sailing he had always assumed.

On a number of occasions, Dominic has told me he's already learning from the experience of having had cancer; the crunch point will come when he has completed his programme of chemotherapy (assuming he doesn't relapse again, which could so easily happen) and is cast adrift, so to speak, after a treatment programme lasting the best part of two years. It's only natural for patients to feel worried and insecure at this point, and I think it's the specialist's job to warn them that this may happen. Assisting patients to ease back gradually into a normal lifestyle is one of the functions, I think, of regular follow-up visits, particularly since the intervals can gradually be stretched and the transition from the 'all or none' phenomenon of total hospital care to 'good luck, you're on your own now' can be greatly softened.

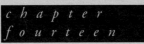

14
chapter fourteen
GYNAECOLOGICAL CANCER

W orldwide, gynaecological cancers form an extremely large and important group of illnesses. In large parts of Asia and South America, cancer of the cervix, for example, is the most important cause of cancer mortality in women, though we know from experience in the developed world that well-run education and screening programmes can reduce the incidence (and therefore the mortality) very substantially. By contrast, the most serious threat in the West comes from ovarian carcinoma, which even now, tends to be diagnosed at a relatively advanced incurable stage, and has a mortality rate equal to the combined mortality rates of cancers of the cervix and uterus combined.

Causes of gynaecological cancer

We know quite a lot about the causes of at least some of the major gynaecological cancers. For example, in cancer of the ovary, women who have never been pregnant clearly have an increased risk of developing the disease; we also know that groups of women with a low incidence, such as the Japanese, do quite rapidly increase their risk if they migrate to a Western society, such as the USA. A striking, fivefold increase seems to occur within a couple of generations, suggesting that environmental influences (rather than genetic ones) are likely to be the cause. Europe and the USA have the largest rates of incidence in the world, and there are certainly a few families reported in which surprisingly large numbers of women with ovarian cancer have been indentified. For the most part, though, it seems to arise sporadically, though there is a weak linkage with breast cancer – possibly operating through the feature of sub-fertility, which is known to be a risk factor in both these conditions.

In cancer of the cervix, there is no doubt that sexual activity is very closely related, and evidence is mounting that the cause of the illness is in some way an infectious virus or particle. A number of studies have shown that the risk of the commonest type of cancer of the cervix (squamous cell carcinoma – see chapter 3) is unknown in nuns and other lifelong celibates. There also seems to be a lowered risk in women who have had one or few sexual partners as opposed to those who have had many, and the risk of disease seems particularly closely related to the age at which a woman's sexual activity first began – the lower the age, the higher the incidence. One explanation may well be that the developing immature epithelium (covering) of the cervix may be particularly susceptible during the immediate post-pubertal years to malign influences, such as a virus particle which might be acquired during intercourse. There are a few cases on record of couples who develop symptoms more or less simultaneously, with the male partner developing a carcinoma of the penis, and within a few years either side, the female partner or spouse developing a carcinoma of the cervix. For many years, it was suggested that women who had intercourse only with circumcised men had a lower incidence of carcinoma of the cervix, but this has been increasingly questioned.

Over the past thirty years, the peak age of incidence of cancer of the cervix has fallen, probably because of changing sexual habits, but the good news is that an increasing proportion of tumours are diagnosed by cervical screening programmes whilst still in the pre-invasive and fully curable stage. There is some evidence that a routine use of a barrier method of contraception (such as a condom) reduces the risk, again supporting the hypothesis that there is a transmissable agent acquired during intercourse which is likely to be the important cause. It is not a simple relationship, however, unlike, for example, the bacteria causing pneumonia or meningitis, or the viruses which cause mumps or chicken pox. The development of a malignant change is a very much slower process, and the causative events much harder to pin down because of the inevitable lag period between initial exposure and development of the disorder. We still do not know which of the virus-type particles is responsible, but the papilloma and herpes viruses have, for many years, been regarded as the main candidates. Some of the herpes viruses, for example, can be shown to produce detectable changes in the microscopic characteristics of human vagina cells, and antibodies to the antigenic components of these viruses are often found in women with cancer of the cervix. Papilloma viruses, on the other hand, are known to cause warts, and genital warts often seem to co-exist with pre-malignant cancer, so these might also be implicated in some way. What is clear, however, is that in patients who are developing a true (invasive) cancer of the cervix, there is a clear development of cellular changes from normality through to an atypical (but not yet malignant) appearance (dysplasia), and then to various degrees of recognisable pre-malignant change (often known as carcinoma-in-situ or CIN).

Not all patients with carcinoma-in-situ will develop an invasive cancer, even without treatment, but a steady slow progression appears to occur in the majority. In countries with well-organised screening programmes, the cervical smear test is designed to make a definitive diagnosis of the abnormalities whilst they are still at this dysplastic or CIN stage, and a regular smear check should certainly give this information, since the two-minute procedure reliably supplies plenty of cells which are fixed directly on the microscope slide, and can then be clearly identified by an experienced cytologist. Early treatment of dysplasia or even severe CIN changes (often referred to as CIN 3, the highest grade) should be one hundred per cent successful. Many of us feel that the present recommendations that cervical screening (often called a Pap smear, after its inventor Dr Papanicolaou) should start early, shortly after a women begins sexual activity, though government guidelines in the UK lag behind this. It is sensible for sexually active women to have a regular smear test every two years, more frequently if dysplastic cells are encountered.

Despite the occasional highly publicised fault in our screening system, there is no doubt that the introduction of screening as a standard part of preventive medicine has led to a dramatic fall in the death rates from cervical cancer. Many cases, particularly in younger women, are now detected earlier at the pre-invasive stage when the disease poses no threat (at least to life, and generally not to fertility either). This is remarkable, since, with increasing evidence of earlier sexual activity, and probably an increased number of partners as well, the stage in post-war Britain (and the West generally) was surely set for an increase in incidence and, by implication, mortality as well. Recent accounts of incompetent technique or false reporting do, however, highlight the need for extreme vigilance at all stages of the screening process.

In carcinoma of the fundus, or body, of the uterus (most commonly an adenocarcinoma, in contrast to cancers of the cervix), there are again wide variations in incidence across the world. It is known, for example, to be very much commoner in Britain and the USA than West Africa, and in general seems to be a disorder of the Western world. It is very much commoner in really overweight women who can genuinely be described as obese (being slightly overweight does not appear to confer any significant risk above normal) and, to a lesser extent, with diabetes and hypertension. The highest rates of incidence in the world are in the USA, where, particularly in urban locations, obesity has become a relatively common health problem. In large ladies with greater then normal fat stores, their normal circulating oestrogen may be supplemented by the conversion of oestrogen precursors in these fat stores, effectively increasing the total circulating oestrogen level, so that stimulation (hyperplasia) of the uterine lining may take place. This development, though not generally associated with malignant change, can, on occasion, develop further, such patients running a well-documented risk of developing cancer. Late menopause also seems to be a clear risk factor, again suggesting a common mechanism, since these patients will have higher oestrogen levels for a longer period than normal.

Which brings us to the question of hormone replacement therapy (HRT). How safe is it? The generally accepted view these days is that modern methods of HRT are extremely safe, since doctors now recommend cyclical oestrogen/progesterone (either by mouth or patches) to mimic as far as possible the normal monthly human cycle. Avoiding over-exposure to high doses of oestrogens (often termed 'unopposed' oestrogens) is an important means of reducing the potential risk of HRT, and there is no doubt that the benefits of HRT (improved well-being and libido together with avoidance of osteoporosis and heart disease) greatly outweigh the potential disadvantages. For patients who have had a hysterectomy, and who are therefore at no risk of developing uterine carcinoma, it is unnecessary to give progesterone-containing forms of HRT. Worries do persist, however, that the very widespread use of HRT, particularly in parts of the US, where many patients are overweight, may lead to an increase in the incidence of uterine hyperplasia, with its theoretical danger of a small risk of development of a malignant change. Certainly it seems sensible to recommend as low a dose of oestrogen as is consistent with the desired symptomatic benefits of HRT, and most manufacturers of HRT preparations now provide more than one dose strength – this applies to both tablets and patches. Recently, concern has been expressed about the possibility that tamoxifen, one of the most valuable and frequently prescribed drugs in breast cancer, may, in a very tiny minority of patients, be causally linked with the later development of endometrial uterine cancer. It was this very concern which delayed the introduction of the long-awaited, and extremely important, tamoxifen prevention study for breast cancer. In my view, however, the enormous benefits of tamoxifen, which is a proven lifesaver for many breast cancer patients, completely outweigh its potential danger.

Fortunately, uterine cancer is one of the most curable forms of all human malignant disease (at least in most cases), but high-risk women (those who are grossly overweight, particularly if they have hypertension or diabetes, and are still menstruating over the age of fifty-three), should certainly be encouraged to lose weight and take proper advice to control the diabetes or high blood pressure as effectively as possible.

Cancers can occur in the lower parts of the female genital tract as well – the vulva and, much less commonly, the vagina. Vulval cancer is almost exclusively a disease of older women, above the age of sixty-five, although exceptions do, of course, occur. As with cancers of the cervix, these are generally squamous cell carcinomas, and this is sometimes preceded, often over many years, by generalised skin changes (again, the term 'dysplastic' is often used, meaning a change in the normal cellular pattern of the skin). Just as with cancer of the cervix, some patients display evidence of carcinoma-in-situ, a pre-invasive condition, prior to the development of the true cancer. Itching, discomfort and occasional surface bleeding are all symptoms of this condition, though it is important to stress that benign causes of these symptoms are very much more common, candida infection, or thrush, being the commonest of all.

Symptoms and diagnosis

The symptoms of gynaecological cancer vary, of course, with the primary site. The lower female genital tract (vulva, vagina and visible part of the cervix) are positioned so low in the pelvis and are so accessible that symptoms often occur relatively early, in sharp contrast to cancers of the ovary. Cancer of the vulva (pretty unusual, only about a thousand new cases occurring annually in Britain) is generally symptomised by itching, pain, a lump on the labia which the patient can feel herself, or a visible ulcer, sometimes with crust and a discharge. Anyone with problems of this type should obviously see their doctor, however embarrassed or sensitive they may be about it. Early treatment is the key to success. If these findings are associated with a lump in the groin area, early treatment is particularly important, since the lump could either be a simple infected gland, or, much more seriously, a malignant lymph node.

Cancer of the cervix is much more common, and the important symptoms are a persistent vaginal discharge, particularly if offensive (smelly) or bloodstained; and pain with intercourse (dyspareunia) or bleeding, particularly after sex. The larger and more locally advanced the tumour, the more obvious these symptoms are likely to be. Unfortunately, some women regard vaginal discharge or intermittent spotting bleeding as a normal feature of their lives, and minimise the symptoms. They should, of course, be taken seriously, particularly since a simple examination and smear test are so easy to perform at the doctor's surgery. Pre-invasive disease (dysplasia and CIN) are not usually associated with symptoms at all, but picked up by routine screening. With uterine cancer, the commonest symptom is post-menopausal bleeding, and any degree of bleeding after the menopause has been reached should be taken seriously – even a single episode! About one-fifth of patients with uterine cancer are pre-menopausal, so bleeding between the periods is also important as a clinical symptom in the younger age group. The symptoms are, of course, even more significant in the high-risk group of overweight patients.

Unfortunately, the symptoms of ovarian cancer are much more nebulous, difficult to pin down and frequently of a non-specific nature. The commonest are lower abdominal pain, bloating, distension and loss of appetite, sometimes with a mild degree of nausea or bowel change. But these are such common symptoms in the normal population anyway that a GP almost has to develop superhuman skills to think of the diagnosis, let alone order the appropriate investigations or make a referral to a specialist on what are likely to seem rather spurious grounds. In truth, the symptoms are remarkably variable – one youngish patient of mine, a Chinese martial arts trainer, was sure that something was wrong after a blow in the lower abdomen from one of her students, which she would normally have parried with ease, caused persistent pain for three weeks – and she was right. She had ovarian cancer and needed urgent surgery and chemotherapy. It is because of the vagueness of these symptoms that many patients are finally diagnosed at a late, and sadly incurable, stage. We badly need new methods of successful screening for ovarian cancer, but our efforts have so far been in vain (more on this later).

Treatment

Patients with gynaecological cancer, or even the suspicion of it, need immediate referral to a specialist, preferably a gynaecologist with an interest in cancer. These specialists are known as gynaecological oncologists, and this whole area is now recognised by the Royal College of Obstetrics and Gynaecologists as an important subspeciality which requires extra training. As with so many branches of surgery, those who perform the operations frequently do, on the whole, produce the best results. Gynaecological cancer is a good example of this, particularly where cancers of the cervix and ovary are concerned, since these are operations requiring special skills not always possessed by every gynaecologist. One of the things the specialist will do is to confirm the diagnosis, by surgical biopsy in the case of accessible cancers – vulva, vagina, cervix – or by dilatation and curettage (D and C, or 'scraping') of the womb, in the case of cancers of the uterus. The dilatation refers to the simple stretching procedure to open up the cervix in order to introduce the proper instrument into the uterus, in order to take samples (curettings) for biopsy purposes. With ovarian cancer, pre-operative biopsy confirmation is not usually possible (or appropriate), but examination and scanning generally give a pretty fair indication of what the diagnosis is likely to be.

Before definitive surgery is considered, it is extremely important to stage patients wherever possible, i.e. gain as detailed an idea of the degree of spread of the cancer as possible, in order to carry out appropriate treatment. Careful staging also allows the treatment results from one centre to be compared with those of another. Increasingly, the staging procedures include the use of computer-assisted or magnetic resonance scans, but more traditional techniques, such as ultrasound and kidney X-rays (often termed IVU – intravenous urogram) are often also helpful. Perhaps most important of all is the EUA – examination under anaesthesia – which will allow the surgeon to inspect, see and feel for him- or herself the degree of local spread of the tumour. With cancers of the vulva and cervix, this may well determine whether or not an operation is the best way forward, or whether the patient might not be better treated with radiotherapy instead. All gynaecological cancers have the potential for spread, and surgery is only likely to be successful with relatively contained tumours – neither the patient nor the surgeon is likely to be very satisfied if an operation is performed with the aim of cure, but the findings on the operating table are more advanced than expected. Careful pre-operative assessment of patients for surgery should cut down on this as far as possible. For vulval and lower vaginal cancers, the commonest routes of spread are to local lymph nodes (generally those in the groin or more deeply within the pelvis), with distant dissemination very unusual indeed. Cancer of the cervix tends to spread both locally, to the supporting structures ('parametrial invasion'), out laterally (sideways) towards the pelvic side wall, and also upwards through lymph node spread. These features are not uncommon in cancer of the cervix, and they usually rule out surgery as a serious option. Radiotherapy is more appropriate in such cases, and may be supplemented by chemotherapy within a clinical trial, since chemotherapy is by no means fully established in this disease, and we urgently need to know whether it can improve survival. Although cancers of the cervix can spread to distant sites, this is fortunately unusual, at least in the early stages of the disease. For the most part, even when patients have such advanced disease that they cannot be cured, the problems are chiefly those of relentless local progression in the pelvis and lower abdomen, rather than distant spread.

With ovarian cancer, the clinical behaviour is altogether different. These tumours certainly do spread widely, though the typical pattern of disease is of involvement throughout the abdominal cavity, sometimes with tumour deposits studding the outside of the bowel or the lining of the abdominal wall, sometimes with the development of tumour fluid (ascites), which often causes abdominal distension. Pre-operative scanning by ultrasound or CT (see chapter 5) often shows evidence of abdominal involvement; a chest X-ray is often done but, fortunately, disease in the chest is unusual.

Once the pre-operative assessment has been completed, treatment can then proceed more logically. If the tumour is well localised, surgery is likely to be recommended, and often offers an excellent chance of cure. No one should underestimate the profound psychological trauma of gynaecological cancer surgery, and no surgeon would recommend a major operation, such as radical hysterectomy (removal of the uterus, cervix, uppermost part of the vagina, supporting structures and more besides) or vulvectomy (removal of the vaginal labia (lips) and surrounding area) without due thought. The latter operation has, fortunately, become more conservative of recent years, and the ever-enlarging role of reconstructive surgery has also helped. With vulvectomy operations, most surgeons feel it best to explore the groin areas to check whether or not the lymph nodes might be affected.

With a radical hysterectomy (often termed a Wertheim hysterectomy, after its originator), the aim, of course, is to eradicate the cancer without any need for additional treatment, such as radiotherapy. It is used for relatively localised invasive cancers of the cervix (these are usually squamous cell carcinomas, but other types of cancer of the cervix are also treated in this same way). If there has been more than minor extension of disease beyond the cervix itself, for example well out towards the pelvic side wall, the operation is usually regarded as being inappropriate, since radiotherapy offers better results, and with surgery, cure becomes impossible with increasing lateral extension of tumour. In point of fact, the results of radiotherapy for early tumours are just as good as surgery, but surgery is generally preferred, particularly in younger, fit women, because the side-effects tend to be less problematic. In the first place, it is usually possible to preserve one or both ovaries surgically, thus retaining the normal hormonal profile (i.e. an endocrinologically pre-menopausal state), whereas with radiotherapy, ovarian irradiation is inevitable, with loss of ovarian function. Secondly, the dose of radiotherapy, although curative, may possibly lead to late side-effects, such as bowel damage or shrinkage of the bladder capacity, which can seriously affect the patient's quality of life. With more advanced cancers, or in patients who are too old or unfit for surgery, there is no choice, radiotherapy offering the only chance of cure.

For uterine cancer, the good news is that most patients are curable by a relatively straightforward hysterectomy (of a less radical variety than the Wertheim hysterectomy), together with removal of the ovaries (most patients are post-menopausal anyway, so removal does not, on the whole, cause much in the way of problems). The majority of these patients don't need further treatment, but those with a significant degree of invasion of the muscular wall of the uterus ('myometrial invasion') are usually recommended to have additional post-operative radiotherapy, either with external methods, or an intravaginal application, or both (see chapter 5). The same applies to patients with other adverse pathological features, notably a severe degree of cellular abnormality – the so-called poorly differentiated cases. By and large, radiotherapy is extremely successful in preventing the development of a local recurrence, the commonest site being the uppermost part of the vagina, where small satellite nodules of disease can otherwise develop.

Radiotherapy for cancer of the cervix is often also remarkably successful, and it is particularly gratifying to be able to cure at least some patients in whom surgical cure was clearly impossible by virtue of local progression of disease or lymph-node involvement. Treatment is likely to be by a combination of external and internal approaches, most centres in the UK now preferring to use external radiation first, and then internal treatment, either by a slow delivery which will involve the patient remaining in hospital (in an isolated room, of course) for up to two or three days; or by the more rapid methods recently introduced, which permit a much higher dose rate, and completion of treatment over two or three minutes. This is often performed under a spinal anaesthetic, and the patient may well be allowed home the same day. An additional advantage of this method is the much greater safety for staff, since the most commonly used equipment is of the remote-control variety, so that the patient can be carefully set into position, with the carrying tubes inserted vaginally, the staff then retiring to an adjacent room to watch the whole procedure on closed-circuit television.

Unfortunately all approaches, whether principally surgical or by radiotherapy, carry a risk of both short and long-term side-effects. For potentially fatal invasive cancer, there really is no other way than to accept a small risk as the possible price of cure. With surgery, the operation has to be radical to be adequate at all; with radiotherapy, the dose has to be high for the best chance of success. Although the risk of severe, late onset side-effects from radiotherapy is not all that great, quite a number of patients do complain of more minor problems, such as persistant loose bowels or intermittent abdominal discomfort. The more severe problems result from scorching of the bowel during the radiotherapy, occasionally to the point where the affected area has to be removed. All radiotherapists know only too well that a high dose, necessary, of course, for successful treatment, is likely to cause this problem in a small minority of patients. It's not easy, though, during the initial consultation, to explain the need for radiotherapy to an extremely anxious patient, newly diagnosed with a potentially life-threatening condition, and with all sorts of personal and family worries to think about, and at the same time to point out in detail the variety of side-effects that the patient may have a very small risk of developing. The degree of information, type of language and the doctor's inclination to provide total reassurance will all vary in each individual case. It's surely right to keep in mind at all times the key objective, namely dealing a death blow to a potentially curable cancer.

In ovarian cancer, surgical removal is extremely important, even in those cases where the tumour has clearly spread beyond the ovary (sadly, the majority), a form of treatment which provides 'debulking' in a way that no other method can quite match. In patients with locally advanced tumours, often involving quite substantial portions of bowel and even the internal aspect of the abdominal wall, it may be necessary for the surgeon to chip away for a lengthy period in order to reduce the tumour bulk down to a level where chemotherapy can then be offered with any real chance of success. Surgical cure of ovarian cancer is certainly achievable, but only in very localised cases, which form no more than twenty per cent of the total group, at best. Fortunately, chemotherapy is of some value in the larger group with more extensive disease, particularly where surgical excision has been possible. Chemotherapy is now given routinely in many cases of ovarian cancer, including all the advanced cases where the patient is fit enough to cope with it (fortunately, the majority). It generally lasts for about six months and is given as intermittent pulses of intravenous therapy, generally every three or four weeks depending on the blood count, most commonly for a total of six courses. There is no definite evidence as to which is the best drug, and trials are in progress to determine this. However, one general point of agreement is that either cisplatin (see chapter 5) or its more recent derivative, carbo-platin, should be used. The main comparative trial taking place in the UK at present is a comparison of carboplatin (given as a single agent) with what was previously regarded as the gold standard – a combina-tion of cisplatin, doxorubicin and cyclophosphamide. The trio of drugs is certainly more toxic; it remains to be seen whether the response rate and overall survival are correspondingly better.

Some patients with ovarian cancer are recommended to have a 'second-look' laparotomy, an operation performed after completion of chemotherapy, to see what has been achieved. The need for a second-look laparotomy is really a recognition that scanning and other methods are not completely able to determine the true state of affairs. The value of this procedure does remain in doubt, though, since some specialists argue that, if residual disease *is* confirmed, there is little more, for the most part, that can be done about it, though I should hasten to add that there are certainly additional anti-cancer drugs available – second line agents – which can be used in these circumstances, and may be valuable, at least in the short term. There is no denying, however, that the presence of residual disease after six courses of chemotherapy is a very unfortunate observation, since long-term survivors are likely to come from the 'no residual disease' group. On the other hand, not all patients are able to undergo the ideal form of debulking surgery prior to chemotherapy; in at least some of these patients, when chemotherapy has really begun to shrink the tumour masses, a second-look laparotomy can be justifiable as a means of attempting to complete a worthwhile operation for the first time. Radiotherapy also has its place in ovarian cancer, but with only a limited role. There are cases, for example, where the chemotherapy has been extremely valuable in clearing upper abdominal disease, but a major bulk of tumour still persists in the pelvis. Pelvic irradiaton can sometimes help to control this, at least for a while.

Most patients who have the right type of surgery for a localised cancer of the cervix, vulva or uterus are cured by it – full stop. In uterine cancer, post-operative treatment with radiotherapy, for those who need it, will cure many more. For surgically incurable patients, treatment of cancer of the cervix by radiotherapy can also be extremely successful, even curative, depending on the stage of disease. Very advanced cases are extremely difficult to cure by any means.

Ovarian cancer is also curable in its early stages, either by surgery or by surgery plus additional chemotherapy, if this is thought advisable. More advanced cases are much more difficult to cure, though many patients live for years if responsive to chemotherapy. These are patients who would almost certainly have been dead within six months of diagnosis and surgery, so chemotherapy is most certainly justifiable, even if unlikely to be curative. With modern supportive care, including highly effective anti-nausea therapy, most patients should get through this treatment without too much difficulty.

Careful follow-up is always needed for patients with gynaecological cancers, ideally in a joint clinic where the gynaecologist and radio-therapist see the patient together and can form a judgement as to the likely outcome. A recent welcome addition has been the recognition that skilled counselling can be extremely helpful in this group – hardly surprising, when you come to think of it. Counselling is so widely used in breast cancer patients that many of the others seem to have been forgotten! In my own hospital, we regularly have counsellors available for patients with gynaecological cancers as well; if anything, I regard them as a more needy group.

In the long term, many patients may well be cured, but with physical or emotional scars that can take years to heal, particularly in younger women, who may have to face not only a life-threatening illness, but also loss of fertility, sexuality and body image. In patients with cancer of the cervix, sex may become more difficult because of the surgical shortening of the vagina or the radiotherapy effect of vaginal dryness and atrophy (thinning of the vaginal lining) from hormonal loss after ovarian irradiation. Hormone replacement therapy (HRT) can certainly be given safely to younger women, and should be offered as a matter of course. It will help to offset many of the problems, but is not enough by itself. These patients need the support of their families, friends and sexual partners and also that of the physicians caring for them, who should do their best to encourage sexual activity (where appropriate) as being both desirable and perfectly safe. Counselling and reassurance are likely to be needed long after the treatment has been completed. Few patients are able simply to 'snap back' into a normal family life when their own has been so disastrously disrupted.

There are some gynaecological cancers, however, in which HRT is ill advised, notably carcinomas of the uterus, in which over-oestrogenisation may have played a part in the initial development of the disease. Many surgeons also feel unhappy about the prospect of giving HRT to patients with glandular cancers of the cervix (adenocarcinoma), since these two may be hormone sensitive. In these patients, a newer form of non-oestrogen HRT (Livial) is probably safer and can be extremely effective. HRT is almost certainly safe in patients who have undergone treatment for ovarian cancer, though conclusive evidence is lacking. Since excess oestrogen production is not regarded as a risk factor for ovarian cancer, there seems no logical reason to avoid it. Unfortunately, a recent multi-centre study designed to test whether or not hormone replacement therapy is safe in ovarian cancer patients looks like failing because of lack of patients suitable for the study. Some of the acute and long-term side-effects of chemotherapy, which these patients may have to face, are described earlier in chapter 5.

There is a very small, but important group of ovarian tumours generally developing in younger patients, and known as teratomas or germ cell tumours, in which chemotherapy is usually curative. These are very similar in nature to the far more common testicular teratoma group, described in chapter 17. Although rare, they are extremely important to diagnose accurately, since they are highly curable, but the correct chemotherapy must be given.

Conclusion

In summary, gynaecological cancers are a very mixed bag. Many are curable, but early diagnosis and treatment are the key. It's always tragic to encounter a patient who could have been cured early on, but a wrong diagnosis, inadequate treatment or, occasionally, the patient's own disinclination to follow medical advice have made this impossible. One still sees the odd patient who follows the 'alternative' path, takes megadoses of vitamins and a highly excluding diet, and falls prey to an unskilled 'healer'. The last such patient I saw was even assured that these methods had led to complete healing of the cancer; no tests, of course – just the certainty of the ignorant. A couple of months later she turned up with obviously advancing disease, finally agreeing to an operation at a time when it was clearly too late. It breaks your heart.

Case history

SARAH'S STORY

Sarah was a stunning redhead of twenty-eight when I first met her. She had first gone to her doctor for a smear test and become concerned when she was recalled. Clearly, the test hadn't been normal, but it looked as though there was no great cause for alarm. It seemed sensible, though, to arrange for a colposcopy, and the gynaecologist was indeed surprised to find a visible abnormality which, of course, he biopsied. This turned out to show the highest grade of cervical pre-cancer (CIN 3), so he arranged for a cone biopsy. Sadly, the biopsy showed not a pre-cancerous, but a true micro-invasive cancer, for which radical hysterectomy would certainly be the correct form of treatment.

Sarah was devastated. It was as if, at each stage, the reassurances she had previously been given proved utterly false; her thoughts, dreams and prayers for motherhood had turned to dust. Worse was to come. At what should have been a curative operation, enlarged glands were noted in the pelvic side wall, subsequently proving, on biopsy, to harbour unexpected metastatic lymph node deposits.

My job was to break the news and explain the need for further treatment which, in my view, should ideally consist of both abdomino-pelvic irradiation and also chemotherapy. We had a long, painful discussion, with tears from Sarah and lame offers of Kleenex from me. 'Will chemotherapy make my hair fall out? Will the radiotherapy dry up my ovaries? Will I be infertile? Could this cancer kill me?' Yes, yes, yes and yes.

You could hardly describe Sarah as lucky, but she did at least have a supportive husband and good friends. After our initial discussion, and a couple more like it to go through the details once again, I had expected her in all probability to decline at least the chemotherapy, but she stuck out her jaw and then her forearm (for the drip) and told me to get on with it.

We're seven years on now, and she and her husband have moved to the country. I still can't quite believe she's cured, but she seems to be, and they've adopted two lovely daughters. I see her just once a year when she comes for her follow-up – always the most gratifying consultation of the day.

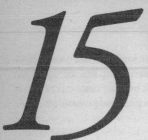

GASTRO-INTESTINAL TUMOURS

The human gastro-intestinal tract is a remarkable and convoluted passageway between mouth and anus (the human fundament, some call it), capable of digesting an astonishing variety of foodstuffs, both nutritious and otherwise, and turning even the most unlikely of substances into a valuable source of energy. Its various components have highly specialised functions; some are compact, such as the mouth and the gall bladder, whereas other sites, notably the small intestine within the abdomen, are lengthy and only contained within the body by ingenious feats of packaging. Although essentially tubular in nature, the gastro-intestinal tract also includes specialised glandular areas, such as the salivary glands, liver and pancreas, whose function is largely to squirt in the appropriate enzymes at differing levels within the pathway, in order to assist the breakdown of foods into components the body can use.

Each of these sites can give rise to cancer, though, oddly enough, the small intestine, the longest by far, very rarely does so. In Western society, the commonest sites for cancer are the mouth (see chapter 21), stomach and large bowel (though not necessarily in that order), although in other parts of the world, primary tumours of the liver or oesophagus are much more common.

It's probably simplest to start at the top and work down.

Oesophageal cancer

Cancer of the oesophagus, or gullet, is usually a male disorder (about two-thirds of all cases), with a peak incidence between the ages of sixty and eighty years. For reasons which are not at all clear, it has increased in incidence over the past decade, and it seems likely that there is a dietary cause (though we don't quite know what is responsible) because of the wide variation in incidence in different parts of the world. In the southern tip of South Africa, for example, it is one of the most common cancers; the same is true in certain parts of Russia and Northern China. In the upper part of the oesophagus, the commonest tumours are squamous cell carcinomas, rather like the tumours of the head and neck region described in chapter 21. As we go down the oesophagus, however, more and more of the tumours are typical adenocarcinomas, indistinguishable from those which are seen in the stomach. These pathological terms are discussed in more detail in chapter 3.

SYMPTOMS AND DIAGNOSIS

The commonest symptom is difficulty in swallowing, often with a sense of the food 'sticking' or lodging at a particular site which is often quite obvious to the patient. As a result, most patients have lost weight – often a considerable amount of weight – by the time they see their doctor and are referred on for specialist advice. There may be very little to detect on general examination, and the key investigation is either a barium swallow test, in which the patient is X-rayed while swallowing a radio-opaque medium containing barium, or direct inspection using a semi-rigid fibre-optic gastroscopy telescope, which allows the oesophagus to be viewed directly. The typical malignant ulcer of oesophageal cancer can often be seen and biopsied quite easily with this latter technique; the barium swallow may give more evidence as to the length of the constriction, since it may not be possible to pass the fibre-optic instrument beyond the constriction which the ulcer so commonly causes, though barium liquid may trickle past and allow quite a decent appreciation of the lengthways anatomy and dimension of the tumour. Even a simple chest X-ray may show whether or not there are glandular nodal enlargements, as a result of the tumour, in the middle of the chest.

TREATMENT

Oesophageal cancer is extremely difficult to deal with. Many patients are in poor shape by the time they come to see the specialist, and the tumour has often spread up and down the cylindrical oesophagus to a substantial degree. Surgical removal is possible only in the minority of cases, and is a very major operation, since lengthy portions of the oesophagus may need to be removed, and either a portion of small bowel or the stomach itself mobilised upwards in order to provide adequate reconstruction. In any event, the long-term results of surgery are not very good, even in this minority of patients who are surgically accessible; for all these reasons, radiotherapy is often preferred as a more realistic method of treatment, which doesn't have immediate mortality (around ten to fifteen per cent) associated with even the best standards of surgical care.

Most patients with oesophageal cancer are not suitable for radical radiotherapy, i.e. radiation given to high dose with the intention of cure. Either they are too unfit, or there might already be evidence of tumour spread to the liver or other sites; or the tumour volume required can simply be too large for the patient to withstand a radical dose. Nonetheless, as with surgery, there are certainly cases on record where even an unpromising carcinoma of the oesophagus has, against all expectation, been cured, though this is unusual. A most welcome advance in the management of oesophageal cancer during the past ten years has been the advent of laser therapy, which has truly transformed the lives of many patients, including those with inoperable disease. The symptomatic effects of oesophageal cancer are mostly the result of direct obstruction of the gullet itself, sometimes to the point where nothing at all can be swallowed, not even the patient's own saliva.

Laser therapy, by burning through the obstruction, can rapidly provide a new channel for the food and liquid to pass through, recanalizing the organ so that decent nutrition can once again be achieved, whilst the patient is considered for additional treatment. Laser therapy is a marvellous means by which the patient can start to eat again, but it is not a fundamental anti-cancer treatment; unlike radiotherapy, it cannot penetrate outside the oesophageal lumen and therefore has no place in the management of the more extensive portion of the tumour, within the wall of the oesophagus itself, or beyond, into the local nodal areas. It is, however, highly complementary with radiotherapy, and the two techniques can be used together. In my view, laser therapy has provided the greatest advance in the symptomatic management of oesophageal cancer over the past twenty years, though overall cure rates remain poor, despite the much-improved palliation that we can now achieve quite regularly. Although radiotherapy is generally given by external beam treatment, the oesophagus lends itself particularly well to the concept of brachytherapy, with the patient swallowing a radio-active tube which can be left in place, sitting snugly against the tumour, for the desired length of time before being removed.

Stomach cancer

Cancers of the stomach have reduced sharply in incidence over the past thirty years, possibly due to improvements in our diet and reduction in smoking rates. Once again, a dietary causation is suggested by the differing rates of prevalence of this tumour in different parts of the world. In Japan, for instance, it is so common that it has become fashionable for normal subjects to have regular screening by fibre-optic direct vision techniques (gastroscopy), every few years. Environmental causes for this tumour are suggested by the fact that Japanese migrants to the United States show a reduction in incidence of the tumour, though still retaining a higher risk than the local indigenous population. The likelihood of developing gastric cancer is also related to social class (possibly through the smoking link), the disease being twice as common in social classes 4 and 5 as in classes 1 and 2.

Although a nutritional or dietary cause of stomach cancer has long been postulated, the nature of the offending substance(s) remains unclear. Certain nitric compounds are known to be dangerous in animals and may also be dangerous in man, and it is widely thought that green vegetables may be protective, possibly by providing high levels of antioxidants which prevent the process of carcinogenesis (cancer-production or development). The same may also be true of vitamin C. It certainly seems clear that a healthy diet, rich in fresh fruit and vegetables and low in dietary fats, offers the best means of avoiding this disease; non-smokers are also known to suffer from it less frequently. The recent excitement about the link between a potentially pathological organism, *Helicobacter Pylori*, and stomach malignancy has once again highlighted the importance of research spanning both the clinic and the lab; it looks as though *H. Pylori* infection may be an extremely important contributor – or even the cause of – stomach cancers, particularly the lymphomatous variety (see chapter 3).

SYMPTOMS AND DIAGNOSIS

Because of the rich lymphatic supply in and around the stomach, the tumour tends to spread early to local intra-abdominal lymph nodes and this, together with early evidence of blood-borne metastasis (most frequently to the liver), makes surgical treatment unsuitable for many patients. The commonest features include abdominal discomfort or ulcer-type symptoms (though one should stress that a benign stomach or duodenal ulcer is far more common than any malignant process), together with lethargy and loss of appetite. Patients often feel bloated, even after a small intake of food, and antacid medications do not generally help the symptoms very much. Quite often, there is a substantial abdominal mass which can be felt by the family doctor or specialist, though this is generally less apparent to the patient himself. If there is evidence of liver involvement, this can also generally be detected in a thorough medical examination. Once again, the important investigations include a barium-meal test and direct inspection using the semi-rigid fibre-optic gastroscope.

TREATMENT

If the growth is limited to a particular part of the stomach, surgical removal ('partial gastrectomy') may be possible, but the larger the tumour, the less likely this is. A total gastrectomy, with complete removal of the stomach, is not often performed, since it has such dire consequences for the patient, the stomach being an organ which is both important and very difficult to reconstruct. On the other hand, patients who have inoperable cancer of the stomach gain very little relief from local radiotherapy, which hasn't much to offer in this condition. This is partly because the stomach is surrounded by so many vital organs that the radiation dose is necessarily limited and partly because of the rather poor intrinsic responsiveness that these tumours seem to display. Chemotherapy is slightly more valuable, perhaps, though there is no clear evidence that early (adjuvant) chemotherapy is helpful in cancers of the stomach, so its use remains limited to symptomatic palliation for inoperable or relapsed cases.

Liver (hepatic) cancer

Primary cancer of the liver is unusual in the Western world, but is very much more common in parts of Africa. The cases we see in Europe arise most frequently in patients with chronic alcoholic damage to the liver (cirrhosis), or where there is evidence of cirrhosis from another cause, such as chronic viral hepatitis.

SYMPTOMS AND DIAGNOSIS

Most patients either have an obvious abdominal mass (generally right-sided) or jaundice, with or without abdominal pain. Many have substantial abdominal distension from the malignant fluid (ascites) produced by the tumour.

Far more common is the development of secondary hepatic (liver) deposits from a primary site elsewhere, most commonly a carcinoma of the large bowel (see page 165). The clinical features tend to be the same as for a primary liver tumour. In both types of hepatic malignancy, blood tests to assess liver function can give a helpful idea as to the likely outcome, though the general outlook is, of course, very gloomy. In patients with secondary liver cancer, the simplest, cheapest and least complicated means of diagnosis is ultrasound scanning, which is both safe, reliable and easily repeated.

TREATMENT

Occasionally, patients with primary cancer of the liver (hepatoma) can be successfully operated on, with removal of the diseased part of the liver. Hepatic transplantation is also gaining ground in these cases, though, as with so many transplant programmes, there is a considerable shortage of organs for donation.

Even with secondary deposits within the liver, it is sometimes possible for the surgeon to remove these if circumstances are favourable, i.e. one or two deposits, in a restricted and accessible part of the organ. On the whole, though, this is not a worthwhile procedure, and treatment with chemotherapy (the details depending on the site of the primary tumour) is more likely to be helpful.

Pancreatic cancer

Pancreatic cancer, a tumour with a very high mortality rate, is unfortunately rising in incidence, though the reasons for this are quite unclear. Interestingly, the time scale of this rise, and its general magnitude, have exactly paralleled the equivalent fall in gastric cancer incidence during the past forty years. It is slightly more prevalent in men, occurring at a peak age of fifty-five to sixty years, and is twice as common in patients with diabetes. It also occurs more frequently in smokers and patients who drink heavily.

SYMPTOMS AND DIAGNOSIS

The majority of these tumours are, once again, adenocarcinomas. Although many people associate the pancreas with insulin production (whose deficiency is the essential cause of diabetes), the main function of the pancreas is not insulin production, but the manufacture of other digestive enzymes which help break down food. Its juices are discharged into the bowel through the pancreatic duct, and it lies in such close apposition to the liver and gall bladder that a tumour in the head of the pancreas (the commonest site) almost always produces jaundice as well as abdominal pain.

TREATMENT

Unfortunately, this generally occurs only at a stage where the tumour is already inoperable by virtue of widespread local extension, both to vital organ and lymph node groups. Surgery is, therefore, of very limited benefit in pancreatic cancer, and, if carried out at all, has to be an operation of almost heroic proportions. Once again, the alternative, regrettably, is of minimal active treatment or the use of radiotherapy (with or without chemotherapy) which is, for the most part, ineffective. Cancers of the pancreas are therefore among the most distressing of tumours, since so little can be done, yet they frequently arise in relatively fit patients below the age of sixty. The outlook is very poor, with radical surgical removal offering the only real hope of cure, and a five-year survival no greater than fifteen per cent. On the other hand, palliative surgery by performing a by-pass between the up- and downstream parts of the bowel can be extremely helpful, even though there is no attempt to remove the tumour itself. By-passing the tumour obstruction does at least improve the symptoms for a period, giving the patient and his family some time to come to terms with the disease. In some patients, it may even be possible to deal with the obstruction without a major operation, by means of an internal 'stenting' procedure, whereby a semi-rigid tube (the stent) is placed into the obstructive duct using a cunning endoscopic approach, passing the instrument all the way down through the oesophagus, stomach, duodenum (the first part of the small bowel) and directly into the blocked area. This extremely ingenious technique is often effective for several months, and at least avoids the very high mortality of more radical surgical procedures for cancers of the pancreas.

Severe unremitting pain can be a real problem with these tumours, but radiotherapy can be helpful in this respect, and proper attention to pain relief with analgesics (pain killers) or nerve blocks can make all the difference.

Bowel cancer

Cancer of the small bowel is fortunately very rare. Less than one in twenty of all gastro-intestinal tumours occur at this site, which seems rather odd, since the small bowel is so lengthy. By contrast, tumours of the large bowel are amongst the most common in the Western world and represent the second largest cause of cancer deaths. The fact that the disease is unusual in large parts of Africa, Asia and South America suggests a possible dietary cause, and there seems little doubt that cancer of the large bowel is far commoner in populations with a high intake of meat products and a relatively low level of dietary fibre. For ten years or so, the evidence has been growing that reducing the intake of meat and animal fat and increasing dietary fibre are both valuable in reducing the incidence of these cancers. Although initially laughed out of court, the surgeon and epidemiologist Sir Denis Burkitt, who initially seemed obsessed with the dietary and bowel habits of rural Africans, was able to show quite clearly that the disease was very unusual in this group, probably because of the rapid rate at which digested food passes through their bowel (the 'increased stool transit time' in medical terminology). This gives far less opportunity for a potential carcinogen to remain in contact with a particular part of the bowel surface for any length of time.

One or two hereditary conditions are also known to predispose to bowel cancer, including the benign but potentially pre-malignant condition of ulcerative colitis, a relapsing large bowel disorder, in which bowel involvement can be extensive. Young patients with this disorder are at particular risk of developing bowel cancer, so much so that, in the past, some physicians recommended total removal of the bowel (total colectomy) in these patients in order to avoid the risk. Nowadays, careful screening and follow-up using fibre-optic colonoscopy has largely replaced this extreme recommendation. In this procedure, a flexible telescope can be introduced at the anus and passed carefully up through the whole of the large bowel, in order to give direct a view and, where necessary, a biopsy of any suspicious site. In familial polyposis, a condition characterised by multiple benign polyps of the bowel, there is also a predisposition to malignant change, particularly in the lower half of the colon, and preventive or 'prophylactic' surgery is sometimes recommended for this group.

Benign (non-familial) polyps of the large bowel are extremely common, and discussion has raged for many years as to whether or not they are genuinely pre-malignant. Bowel polyps are discovered increasingly with advancing age, and only a small percentage will become malignant, though evidence of a previously benign-looking polyp is sometimes found close by the malignant tumour in the surgical specimen, raising the question of whether or not an originally benign polyp might have become a more aggressive tumour. It certainly seems clear that large polyps carry a greater risk than smaller ones and that there is a particular variety of benign tumour, the villous adenoma of the lowest part of the large bowel (the rectum), which is genuinely pre-malignant, and should be removed.

SYMPTOMS AND DIAGNOSIS

Most patients with cancer of the bowel have a fairly obvious change in bowel habit, i.e. constipation and/or diarrhoea. Quite often, these rather unusual tumours are symptomised by a watery discharge from the rectum, rather than obstruction and pain. The precise position of the tumour within the large bowel often dictates the nature of other symptoms such as pain, rectal bleeding or weight loss. Tumours of the right side (ascending colon) tend to cause more in the way of abdominal pain than left-sided (descending colon) or rectal tumours, whereas, perhaps not surprisingly, cancers of the rectum present far more commonly with bleeding. Complete obstruction, with inability to open the bowels at all (and often with persistent vomiting and discomfort) occurs in about ten per cent of cases, and abdominal pain is more common with colonic than rectal cancers. Rectal bleeding may be obvious, with fresh, bright-red blood mixed into the stool, but tumours from higher up the bowel are more likely to cause 'melaena' or black stools, because the blood has become denatured by the time it appears in the expelled stools. The pain of colonic cancer is typically colicky, coming and going, intermittent, sometimes rising to a very severe cramp-like crescendo.

These symptoms require urgent attention and evaluation. A rectal examination by the family doctor or specialist will often be sufficient to suggest the diagnosis in rectal cancers, though obviously, tumours higher in the bowel are well beyond the reach of the examining finger. Early referral to an abdominal surgeon is extremely important, and patients should never be expected to wait, since early detection and treatment is the key to success for large bowel cancer.

The investigations will almost certainly include a sigmoidoscopy, which is the insertion of a rigid tube, with proper illumination and biopsy attachments, into the rectum and lowest part of the colon itself (the sigmoid colon, situated towards the left side of the lower abdomen). This gives rapid diagnosis in a large proportion of colorectal tumours, since well over half of all large bowel cancer in the Western world are situated in the rectum or sigmoid – again, suggesting that food carcinogens are the cause of these tumours, since this part of the bowel is the final depot for digested food particles before expulsion. Other important investigations include the barium enema, in which a tube is inserted into the anus and radio-opaque barium dye passed as a liquid up into the bowel. This is an excellent technique which gives good radiographic images of the whole of the large bowel, i.e. well beyond the reach of the sigmoidoscope, and the investigation may give sufficient information about the position of a probable cancer for the surgeon to perform the appropriate operation without further ado. The bowel must be carefully cleaned and prepared before a barium enema procedure, which may involve a fair degree of discomfort from the laxatives which are used. The quality of the pictures, however, does justify this undignified performance. Many surgeons will also wish to see a CT scan of the pelvis and lower abdomen, in order to check whether there is evidence of disease outside the bowel, a most important feature of some bowel cancers which may limit their operability and make non-surgical treatment more appropriate.

TREATMENT

Most of the large bowel tumours are typical adenocarcinomas, and the important pathological features are the degree of invasion from the inside of the bowel wall (the mucosa or lining) through the muscular coating of the bowel to the outer surface (the serosa), and whether or not the surgeon and pathologist find evidence of lymph-node involvement in the resected bowel specimen. This type of surgical staging has stood the test of time and is known to be the most important indicator of outcome. Most patients with early-stage bowel cancers, confined to the mucosa, are cured by the appropriate operation, though surgeons generally prefer to remove a generous portion of bowel in order to make sure that the margins of clearance are sufficiently generous. Cancers of the ascending colon are often dealt with by a right hemicolectomy (essentially removing the whole of the right-hand portion of the large bowel), and tumours of the descending and upper sigmoid colon by a left hemicolectomy (the same, but on the left side). Fortunately, there is sufficient redundancy in the human intestine that we can do perfectly well with only half the large bowel; the operations just mentioned generally result in an excellent outcome, with careful anastomosis (joining-up) of the cut ends of the bowel, and no permanent need for a colostomy.

Cancers of the lower bowel, however, including many rectal carcinomas, will generally require either a temporary or permanent colostomy, in which the upper (proximal) cut end of the bowel is brought out on to the abdominal wall, with a stoma and a collecting bag for the faeces, rather than attempting a dangerous anastomosis at the lowest rectal or anal level, for fear that the operation will be insufficiently generous to clear the cancer completely. Obviously, it is always extremely disappointing for patients to hear that they may have to have a colostomy procedure, but for many, it will be the price of a permanent cure. Although many patients are naturally worried about the appearance of a colostomy and the possibility of constant embarrassment, social isolation, spillage and smell, most are also worried that they will find it impossible to manage the colostomy themselves without skilled help. They need encouragement, support and reassurance that the presence of the colostomy does not imply that part of the cancer has been left behind, or that it will prove impossible to return to a normal active life. Many patients faced with the possibility of a permanent colostomy find it extremely helpful to meet others who have undergone this procedure and have learned to cope with it before facing surgery themselves. They, in turn, are then sometimes called on to counsel other patients, and may gain considerable self-esteem from making this contribution to the welfare of others. Although some patients take many months to come to terms with a colostomy, the majority find it far less difficult and degrading than they might have expected. Large hospitals have stoma therapy staff, often with a nursing background, who are able to educate, counsel and support patients with colostomies. Self-help groups, such as the Colostomy Welfare Association, are also extremely active in this field.

Tumours which have penetrated a significant portion of the bowel musculature, or have broken through to the outside or to local lymph nodes, are much more difficult to control by surgery alone. Fortunately, it has become increasingly clear over the past ten years that both chemotherapy and radiotherapy have a part to play. Early (adjuvant) use of chemotherapy, i.e. immediately after surgery, without waiting for a recurrence, can improve the outcome in these more advanced tumours, even though the additional benefit may be rather limited at present, since currently available anti-cancer agents are not especially powerful in bowel cancer. The value of additional, post-operative radiotherapy for locally advanced large bowel cancers is limited to rectal tumours, but can be extremely valuable from the point of view of preventing a local recurrence. It is this danger, together with the risk of more widespread involvement (particularly to the liver), that represents the greatest threat to the health of a patient who has successfully undergone surgery for cancer of the bowel.

The possibility of tumour recurrence at the site of the anastomosis is a particular worry, so abdominal surgeons take particular care to avoid tumour spillage during operations, and to achieve safe margins – hence the lengthy portion of bowel that is often removed in surgery. As for metastatic involvement to the liver, it is a curious fact that this unwelcome eventuality, though always regrettable, does not always imply rapid progression and early death. For some reason, a proportion of patients with liver deposits from rectal or colonic carcinomas can live for many months or even years with the appropriate treatment – generally chemotherapy, but, just occasionally, surgical removal of the secondary deposits or laser therapy (still an experimental technique) if limited to a particular part of the liver.

Over eighty per cent of patients with early carcinomas, confined to the mucosa, survive for five years, and the majority of these patients prove, in the long run, to have been completely cured by surgery. Where there has been involvement of the muscle of the bowel wall, the figure falls to about fifty per cent. Even lymph node involvement can be associated with lengthy survival and probable cure if the nodes have all been resected. In these more adverse cases, the surgeon is likely to discuss the possible need for chemotherapy and/or radiotherapy, but, if not, patients should not feel shy about asking the surgeon's view about these potential forms of treatment. There is certainly no doubt that surgery remains the absolute cornerstone of treatment – radiotherapy or chemotherapy, though extremely valuable in certain cases, will not be replacing surgery altogether in the foreseeable future.

Bowel cancers at the lowest level of all, the anus, have increased in frequency during recent years, though they still only account for a tiny minority of large bowel cancers. Until a few years ago, anal cancer was slightly more common in women, but it appears to be an AIDS-related malignancy and certainly became more common in gay men during the 1980s. It is generally treated by radiotherapy (with or without chemotherapy – there is an excellent UK randomised trial on this which has just been successfully completed) in order to preserve the anal sphincter and, as far as possible, normal bowel functioning without colostomy. A few cases, however, are too large for radiotherapy to be possible, and surgical resection, which always requires colostomy, may be required for a small proportion of these patients. It is worth stressing, however, that, only a few years ago, all patients with anal cancer were recommended to have this type of surgery, so this welcome change towards non-surgical treatment does represent a real step in the right direction. In the recent UK trial just mentioned, the combination of radiotherapy and chemotherapy proved so successful – compared to radiotherapy alone – that this form of treatment should now be regarded as standard therapy. We can now say with confidence that there is a smaller probability of a colostomy being required, as a result of failure of control at the primary site, with the combination. An enormous step forward, most would agree – but only because the right clinical trial was performed.

Large bowel tumours do sometimes produce a tumour marker known as CEA (carcino-embryonic antigen) which, although not specific to bowel cancer, can be a very valuable means of following the progress of the tumour. Such markers can be used to identify a probable recurrence before the patient had developed symptoms, while it is still likely to be surgically removable. It's not yet entirely clear whether the routine use of CEA monitoring will definitely improve survival results; this is another area of current study by a randomised controlled trial. Watch this space, as they say.

Case histories

MILDRED'S STORY

Mildred had been constipated for as long as she could remember, but couldn't ever recall it being quite this bad. Divorced ten years previously, and now aged seventy-one, she had struggled to get her life back together after a rather bitter marriage lasting almost thirty years and producing two extremely dislikeable children; despite her positive, no-nonsense approach to life, she was, in truth, shut off from her family and the rest of the world around her.

She was embarrassed to go to her GP, but felt she had to. The GP thought she could feel something odd with the tip of her examining finger, so she sent Mildred off to the local specialist, who saw her after a six-week gap. By this time, the rectal carcinoma was a little bigger, and the surgeon had no difficulty confirming its presence with a sigmoid-oscopy and barium enema. She was hopeful that it could be resected without the need for a permanent colostomy.

In the event, Mildred was relatively lucky and no permanent colostomy was needed, but unfortunately that wasn't the end of the matter. Although the surgeon had found no evidence of tumour dissemination within the abdomen, the pathologist later confirmed that there was, indeed, significant evidence of spread through the bowel wall and explained as much to her surgical colleague at their monthly conference, with the slides projected onto a screen. The surgeon sought the opinion of the radiotherapist, since surgery alone was clearly not very likely to cure the patient.

The radiotherapist explained the wide variety of opinion, but said that, in her own view, the sensible course of action would be to have both radiotherapy and chemotherapy, 'to be on the safe side'. Mildred did extremely well with this treatment, although the painful skin reaction, particularly between her buttocks, was more uncomfortable than she had bargained for. Most of the staff had warned her that the chemotherapy was likely to be worse, but, with her, it was the other way round.

Eighteen months later, they told her that one of the blood tests they had been using to monitor her progress had shown a slight rise in one of the marker levels (it was the CEA test) and a further scan would have to be done. Sadly, this showed evidence of two small secondary cancer deposits within the liver, and these would have to be dealt with by laser, surgery or chemotherapy. Mildred was reasonably happy to leave the decision to the experts, and, in the end, a combination of all three techniques was felt to offer the best chance of success.

Twelve months on, she has now completed the whole of the planned treatment, all of which went well. In the end, she lost about a third of her liver, leaving her quite sufficient to get by on, and she's now been off treatment for six months with no evidence of a further rise in the CEA. In the meantime, Mildred seems to have blossomed in a curious sort of way. Previously, she was rather tied to her home, but having now decided that one of her two children isn't quite as unappealing as she had thought, having done the decent thing and produced two grandchildren for her to inspect, she took herself off to visit them in Australia last month. She'd never flown before, but the postcard tells me she arrived safely. What pleases me most is the control she's beginning to take over her own affairs. On the bottom of the card, it said, 'The specialist you referred me to at St P's, Melbourne, told me he doesn't routinely do CEA tests. I told him I've never heard such nonsense. Please fax details of another specialist.'

ALBERT'S STORY

Albert was fifty-six when his symptoms began, fifty-eight when cancer of the pancreas was diagnosed and fifty-nine when he died. He had noticed back pain for a month or two, but was a stoical sort of fellow and simply put up with it. His wife badgered him to see the doctor, but he wasn't keen. 'Indigestion,' he said.

However, after three more weeks of sleepless nights with Albert propped up in bed and clearly losing weight, she lost patience and got the GP round. Albert wasn't at all pleased and, out of spite, deliberately dropped cigarette ash over the bedclothes. The doctor was worried, but couldn't examine Albert properly, as he was too ill to move. The GP therefore arranged for a home visit by the local physician (hospital specialist). He was also worried. 'Look at it this way, Albert,' he said, 'If it really is indigestion, it's pretty severe and hasn't responded to antacids and Tagamet; if it's just back pain, it would have got better by now; if it's something really serious, the sooner we know, the better.'

That really did scare Albert, but he was a stubborn man and only agreed to go into hospital after another week of relentless pleading by his wife. In hospital, the physician's suspicions were strengthened; he hadn't been able to examine Albert properly at home, but it was easier in the hospital bed, and he was in little doubt that he could feel a firm abdominal mass. A CT scan and a needle biopsy confirmed his suspicions – cancer of the pancreas. As with most cases, it was clearly inoperable, at least from the point of view of total tumour resection, by virtue of its close association with unresectable surrounding structures. 'Not good news, I'm afraid,' said the surgeon. 'Perhaps I'd be better off at home, then,' said Albert.

On the morning of his planned discharge three days later, when the pain was finally under control with regular, long-acting morphine, they noticed for the first time a tinge of jaundice. By the time of Albert's first follow-up visit two weeks later, the jaundice was obvious to all. 'I'm afraid we'll have to get you back in to do a by-pass,' said the surgeon. 'If you want to do an operation, why didn't you do it first time around?' asked Albert. A further three weeks went by, the jaundice deepening almost every day, before he agreed to be re-admitted. By this time, the pain had become more severe, despite the long-acting morphine, and the Macmillan Support Network had been called in by his GP. Perhaps it was too late.

As it turned out, the operation was rather more of a success than anyone had dared hope. Albert had become so itchy with the jaundice that it was more than just a cosmetic relief when it started to clear within days of the operation. The Macmillan team supervised the pain control with expert efficiency, and just over two weeks later, he was at home with his wife. He knew he was going to die, of course, but it took longer than expected. They'd all wanted him to die at home, though eventually his wife had her doubts – she just wasn't sure whether she'd cope or not, even with the help available. 'I keep trying to imagine what it'll be like at the end, but I can't quite manage it.' 'You'll cope, don't worry, you'll cope,' said the Macmillan nurse.

Albert's wife was magnificent. She turned out to be more of a coper than she had dreamed possible. Most of the time, the Macmillan team stayed in the background, but it was good to know that they were always there. She and Albert hadn't been great talkers, but suddenly they found themselves more in tune than before. He wasn't a religious man, he said, but he wanted to get a few things off his chest. 'He actually apologised to me for all that f'ing and blinding when he used to go out drinking,' she told me later, after he had died. 'I was angry with him for bringing that up when the truth was far worse – women, gambling, the lot. But I suppose I loved him all the same – and I was pleased I could look after him until the end.'

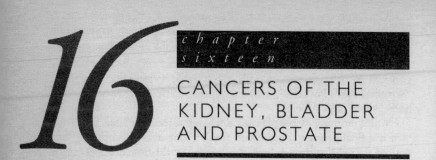

16

CANCERS OF THE KIDNEY, BLADDER AND PROSTATE

T hese, too, are a mixed bag, accounting for over a quarter of all cancers in men. Within this group, renal (kidney) tumours are by far the least common.

Causes of renal, bladder and prostate cancers

As far as causation is concerned, we have only a few rather sketchy clues. Both renal and bladder tumours are more prevalent in smokers or ex-smokers and are commoner in men (about three to one for cancers of the kidney and about six to one for bladder cancer). For tumours of the kidney, there is at least one congenital syndrome (a curious disease known as von Hippel-Lindau syndrome), characterised by spongy blood vessel overgrowths (haemangioblastomas) in parts of the brain, in which, for some reason, it happens to be quite common. In the outflow part of the kidney, the collecting system, tumours occur which are different in type from the commonest variety (adenocarcinoma). In these less common types, there is sometimes a history of kidney stone formation.

For bladder cancers, we know rather more about causation. By the end of the nineteenth century, it was recognised that workers in the aniline dye industry had a higher incidence of this type of cancer than expected, and it later became clear that this was due to a carcinogen, a cancer-promoting substance, produced during the dye-production process. Other occupational groups have been recognised, notably those in the rubber and cable industries. Bladder cancer is also reportedly more common in urban than rural areas, and one other important predisposing feature, of great significance in the Middle East, is the importance of chronic bladder infection in predisposing patients to malignant change. The most important of these infections is schistosomiasis, caused by a burrowing fluke which chronically infests the bladder wall, entering the body by a direct, water-borne route, chiefly from polluted rivers or streams. As for cancer of the prostate, very little is known about its causation, though it is among the commonest of all male cancers, increasing in incidence directly with advancing age. It is even thought possible that all men who live long enough will develop it, though not necessarily as a clinical problem during life. In the United States, it is the third commonest cause of cancer death in males, exceeded only by lung and large bowel cancers. US figures also show a much higher mortality rate in blacks than whites, and it is one of the malignancies which appears to have become more common over the past fifty years. It is clearly hormone dependent and doesn't occur in men who have been castrated.

The kidneys are situated on either side of the mid-abdomen, the right slightly lower than the left and fairly far back (posteriorly) on either side of the spinal column. They are supplied with blood by the renal artery, and each makes urine separately, passing it down through a collecting system and ureter, each of which passes downwards through the abdomen, connecting with the bladder, in which urine is stored. Its final path is via the urethra, which travels through the penis in men and more directly to the lowest part of the vagina in women. Cancers of the ureter and urethra are extremely uncommon, and those of the penis are unusual as well.

Symptoms and diagnosis

As far as symptoms are concerned, they are, of course, likely to be related to the formation and passage of urine. In both kidney and bladder tumours, the commonest symptom is haematuria, or bleeding into the urine. In bladder cancer, this is generally painless, though many patients have symptoms such as urgency of micturition (a very strong desire to pass urine), nocturia (passing urine at night) and frequency of micturition or reduction of the urinary stream. In cancer of the kidney, pain is more often a feature, though even large kidney tumours can be surprisingly painless. Occasionally, the patient will notice a mass in the loin area himself. However, with cancer of the prostate, the discovery of the malignant tumour is usually an incidental finding at surgery for what was thought to be a benign prostatic enlargement – or, more accurately, after surgery, when the pathology report is available. Many elderly men require such surgery because enlargement of the prostate (far more commonly a benign than a malignant disorder) has caused obstruction of the urethra, producing difficulties with micturition as described above. It is often possible, though, to detect a prostate cancer simply by rectal examination, since a watchful doctor can recognise that the prostate gland, which can be felt quite easily, often feels hard or craggy if there are malignant changes within it. A significant proportion of the patients with prostatic cancer do, however, have symptoms of secondary spread, since this is relatively common, chiefly affecting the bones of the pelvis, hips and lower vertebral area. To some extent, this also applies to the far less commonly encountered cancers of the kidney, since these also metastasise to bone.

Treatment

Although patients with frequency of micturition and discomfort may simply be suffering from cystitis, persistent symptoms will require investigation, and an urgent appointment with a urologist should be sought. If examination reveals an obvious loin mass, the quickest confirmatory test is usually an ultrasound of the kidney, followed by a CT or MRI scan. In most patients with haematuria, the urologist will arrange for cystoscopy, a simple and extremely informative investigation in which a narrow tube (cystoscope) is passed directly through the penis into the bladder, giving very good direct vision of the whole of the bladder's interior surface. This will often reveal one or more areas of tumour; in some cases, a substantial portion of the bladder mucosa (lining) is involved. Cystoscopic biopsy will also reveal the extent to which the tumour has penetrated from the bladder lining into the muscular wall, a most important pathological feature with considerable prognostic weight. For relatively superficial tumours within the bladder, the use of local heat application (cystodiathermy) to burn the tumours away is often very effective, but may have to be repeated on a number of occasions. If the tumours are larger or more extensive, chemotherapy can be given directly into the bladder, again on repeated occasions. In any event, virtually all patients with bladder cancer require repeat cystoscopy at regular intervals, in order to monitor progress. This is generally done under a short anaesthetic as a day case.

For more deeply situated bladder tumours which invade the muscular wall, the risk of dissemination to other parts of the body (local lymph nodes, lung, liver and bone) is considerably greater, and cystodiathermy and intravesical chemotherapy (i.e. direct instillation into the bladder) are insufficient. Either radiotherapy or cystectomy (removal of the bladder) will be necessary. Both are effective, but, not surprisingly, treatment by radical radiotherapy has become more widely employed since it was recognised as a valuable treatment in the 1950s, as few patients would willingly lose their bladder, with the inevitable consequence of requiring a new route for urine flow – generally achieved by means of an ileal conduit, formed from a short portion of bowel, with the ureters implanted directly into it and brought out on to the abdominal wall with a permanent stoma and collecting bag. Radical radiotherapy for deeply penetrating bladder tumours is frequently very effective, although a cure can never be guaranteed. It may be slightly less successful than total cystectomy, but with the enormous advantage of preservation of the bladder. If a local recurrence does occur, it is generally possible to consider total cystectomy at a later stage. The question is often asked whether or not the cure can be achieved by partial bladder removal, with reconstruction of the remainder to form a smaller, but still reasonably adequate bladder. Few bladder tumours are treatable in this way, partly because the disease is often quite widespread within the bladder and, in any event, the whole of the bladder lining is often unstable in these patients. By and large, the treatment of deeply invading bladder cancer lies between radical radiotherapy and radical surgery. If patients are to be considered for either form of treatment, pelvic scanning is essential to determine the limits of the tumour, since, not uncommonly, evidence of extra-vesical spread (i.e. outside the bladder) will be discovered.

Although most patients are happier with the prospect of facing radical radiotherapy rather than surgery, the treatment course can be quite arduous. It lasts between three and six weeks, depending on local practice, and may produce quite uncomfortable urinary symptoms as a result of the direct effect of the X-ray beam on the bladder lining. Urinary frequency and nocturia are among the more problematic of these symptoms, in many patients persisting long after the course of treatment. Repeat cystoscopy will be required in all cases to ascertain whether or not the treatment has been successful; in some patients, the radiotherapy appears to shrink the bladder permanently, so that they have to accept the probability of more frequent micturition (including at night) as a long-term consequence of cure.

For more superficially placed tumours, new treatments are coming in all the time. Apart from cystodiathermy, cryosurgery (treatment by extreme freezing) and laser are also possible, and the range of suitable intra-vesical therapy agents has grown rapidly over the past few years. Instillation of BCG (the agent often used to immunise against tuberculosis during childhood) directly into the bladder is also effective in slowing down the rate of progression of these tumours.

Cancers of the penis are uncommon. They tend to develop near the tip of the penis rather than the shaft, sometimes with a very slow period of evolution, over many years. In appearance, they may resemble an ulcer – though non-malignant ulcers are far more common! They tend to spread to the nodes in the groin (the inguinal area) and are treated either by radiotheraphy or surgery, sometimes both. Usually they are fairly well localised, and, understandably, most patients prefer radiotherapy, which can often produce an excellent result with full healing and no further problems. Surgery will be necessary, however, if the patient suffers a local recurrence; fortunately, it is often possible to perform local surgery, without having to amputate the whole organ. Half a penis can work surprisingly well. The worrying feature of penile cancer is that, if it has spread to the inguinal and other nodal areas, cure is much more difficult. Cancer of the penis often seems to run a slow, rather indolent course, with some patients appearing cured by the initial radiotherapy, but developing a local recurrence or inguinal lymph node disease many years after initial treatment.

Cancers of the kidney should be dealt with by surgery if at all possible. We only need one kidney, so it is perfectly feasible and technically correct to remove the whole of the kidney (nephrectomy) if a renal cancer is discovered. The ureter is often removed as well (and is certainly not much use anyway, without the kidney). Although this may cure the cancer, some renal tumours are locally very advanced and cure cannot be guaranteed, even with removal of the whole kidney. These tumours do also have a reputation for late dissemination, notably to bone and lung, so careful follow-up is important. In patients who have evidence of widespread disease, even at diagnosis, nephrectomy may still be a sensible approach if the primary tumour is causing real discomfort or other symptoms. There are even cases on record in which removal of the primary tumour has resulted in shrinkage of the other deposits, though we still do not know why this occasionally occurs. It's not very common, but every cancer specialist knows another who says a friend of his has seen it on one or two occasions! An alternative is to 'embolise' the tumour, a technique which was devised a few years ago, with the specific intent of trying to shrink the tumour down by interrupting its blood supply with an injection of material with occlusive properties, directly into the renal artery, which gives the kidney its blood supply.

For cancer of the prostate, generally an adenocarcinoma, tumour staging is again important, since this is likely to dictate treatment as well as determine outcome. Ultrasound techniques have become highly sophisticated, with direct scanning of the prostate possible by means of the trans-rectal route, since the scanner tip can then be placed in almost direct proximity to the prostate itself, separated only by a centimetre or so. In patients who seem likely to have a prostatic carcinoma detected before a trans-urethral resection procedure (TUR), prostatic biopsy using the trans-rectal route can easily be accomplished with minimal anaethesia. As with bladder cancer, CT and MRI scanning will give important information as to the local extent of disease.

As far as the management is concerned, there are few areas in cancer where such diversity of opinion exists, even among experts. There is not even complete agreement that early localised treatment of prostatic cancer should be undertaken by local means (surgery or radiotherapy) at all, though most would agree that some attempt at curative therapy should be made. One alternative, hotly debated among urologists and urological cancer specialists, is the use of hormone treatments, since it has been known for over fifty years that most prostatic cancers are hormonally dependent. Both oestrogen therapy (female hormones) and orchidectomy (removal of both testicles) have been known for many decades to be useful for palliation, often benefiting patients who have widespread, painful bone disease from secondary prostate cancer. Since many patients, including all those with a positive bone scan diagnosis, are unsuitable for radical surgery or radiotherapy, the use of these (and newer) hormone techniques – see below – has become increasingly routine, as part of standard therapy both for early and advanced cases.

In patients with localised disease, radical radiation therapy is generally preferred as the treatment of choice, and surgery (radical prostatectomy) has largely been dropped. As with radical irradiation for bladder cancers, symptoms during and after prostatic radiation can be quite troublesome, though the non-malignant part of the prostate itself does appear to tolerate radiotherapy very well. This form of treatment is extremely effective for early, well-localised tumours, with many patients retaining normal bladder functioning and sexual potency afterwards, unless adjuvant hormone therapy has also been recommended, in an attempt to reduce the male hormone (testosterone) levels to zero. For patients with more advanced disease, where there is no prospect of cure, hormone treatments clearly offer the best chance of long-term palliation, and there are many agents available, of which the most commonly used nowadays are probably cyproterone (given in tablet form) and the more recently introduced goserelin, given as a monthly injection.

The mechanism of action of these agents is quite different – they work by reducing testosterone levels via an effect of the pituitary gland at the base of the brain – and they have replaced the old-fashioned approach with oestrogen tablets, which used to cause undesirable feminisation, quite often including breast enlargement. In some cases, though, treatment by orchidectomy (removal of the testicles) is the only means of gaining control of the tumour. Not, of course, a step which would ever be undertaken lightly but often accepted by these predominantly, elderly patients extremely well. As far as treatment results are concerned, it is difficult to assess results in prostate cancer because of its uncertain and often slow natural history, and the high death rate in any group of elderly men. Although true cure is unusual, with patients continuing to relapse several years after treatment, about fifty per cent of patients are alive after ten years, and with better results in patients where the disease was apparently limited to the prostate gland without evidence of local extension to sites just beyond. Few patients with bone deposits survive in the long term, despite high initial response rates to hormone therapy, and chemotherapy has remained consistently disappointing as a potential additional method of treatment.

It is important to stress that treatment of these urological malignancies can be fully consistent with a remarkably normal quality of life. The many competing treatments now available – including surgery, radiotherapy, chemotherapy (particularly in bladder cancer, in which it is now much more widely used) and, in the case of prostate cancer, hormone therapy – mean that many patients have to find their way through quite a complex treatment maze. Although many are in late middle age or beyond, age *per se* should never be a reason to compromise treatment intensity, particularly where cure is a realistic possibility.

Case history

RICHARD'S STORY

Richard had just turned fifty when he developed low back pain and weakness of the legs. He saw his doctor, who said it was a disc and laid him off work for a fortnight. However, as a self-employed travelling salesman, it was costing him money and, in any event, he wasn't much better after a week, so he simply got on with his life and took Nurofen for the pain.

A month later, he collapsed in the street when his legs buckled under him, and a passing cab driver brought him into our casualty department, where an X-ray confirmed almost total destruction of the lowest two lumbar vertebrae. There was no clue as to what might be the cause, and general examination was normal apart from his grossly weakened legs, so a biopsy was performed by one of the orthopaedic surgeons.

A week later, the pathologists reported undoubted malignancy, but they were quite certain that the lumbar vertebrae were a secondary rather than the primary site, since the microscopic appearances didn't correspond to any of the known primary cancers of the bone. Could this be a cancer of the kidney, they wondered? Sure enough, the abdominal ultrasound confirmed a substantial primary cancer of the right kidney, measuring almost 10 centimetres across, which, despite its size, had not previously declared itself. I'd already done an isotope bone scan, and no other secondary deposits were seen.

It was clear that Richard ought to have a course of palliative radiotherapy to the lower spine, and, fortunately, his pain improved a good deal, although he still required the long-acting morphine tablets we had prescribed after the diagnosis had first been made. Radiotherapy reduced his morphine requirement by about two-thirds. I thought it might just be worthwhile asking a urologist to see him, in case there was any advantage in removing the kidney, but, at the end of the day, he thought not, so radiotherapy is the only form of active treatment Richard has had.

Eighteen months have now gone by, and he's doing pretty well. The real problem, though, is that, despite his happy-go-lucky character, his wife simply can't cope with the uncertainty of it all. Although not burdened with guilt about her own good health and his infirmity (as many are), she's constantly close to the edge with a degree of anxiety that rarely leaves her alone; counselling hasn't really helped. For Richard, struggling on gamely with an incurable disease currently under control, her inability to support him (or even cope with her own distress) is the most exhausting aspect of the illness. He feels somewhat cheated to have discovered that he, the patient with the illness, is expected to be the strong one. Clearly, he finds it easier to cope with the uncertainty and lack of additional treatment than his wife does, and my best hope is that, despite her anxiety, further counselling will help her to develop the sensitivity and skill she needs in order to learn how to stop driving him crazy with her constant, well-meant attentions and cross-questioning.

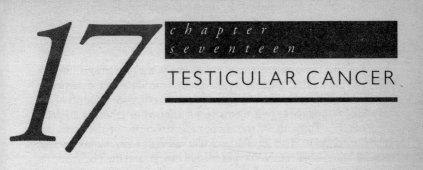

17

chapter
seventeen

TESTICULAR CANCER

Causes of testicular cancer

Testicular tumours have certainly become more common over the past twenty years, though no one quite knows why. We certainly know one or two important predisposing factors, though, of which the most consistent is the presence of an undescended testicle, a congenital abnormality which some boys are born with and which confers an increasing risk of malignant change of the testes the longer it is left in its incorrect position – generally in the abdomen or in the inguinal (groin) region. Before birth, the testicles are situated within the abdomen and pass through the inguinal canal to their final position, and it may well be that the additional warmth of the abdominal environment is the stimulating factor in provoking malignant change, since the normal testicle is, of course, subject to a much lower temperature, effectively outside the body within the scrotum. Interestingly, in boys who have a single undescended testicle, it is not only this one, but the other, too, which is at increased risk of cancer in later life, so it really is of the utmost importance to perform a surgical correction of an undescended testis. There is a second reason, too: poorly descended testicles rarely produce sperm, so relative infertility or subfertility is another likely consequence. Trauma to the testes is often implicated as a causative factor for cancer, but this is generally believed (by the medical profession, at any rate) to be untrue. However, there may be more to the suggestion that inflammation of the testes during a mumps episode (so-called mumps orchitis) may predispose to testicular malignancy.

Symptoms and diagnosis

Most testicular tumours are termed either seminoma or teratoma (though much more complicated terms are also used) depending on the particular type of malignancy, but the important fact is that they are tumours of the potentially reproductive cells themselves – referred to generally as 'germ cell tumours'. Tumours of the supporting structures of the testes are much less common. This sets the testicular tumours apart, pathologically, from the other more common types of solid cancer, and their behaviour is very different too. Although they spread by the classical pathways of blood-borne, lymphatic and direct local extension, their response to radiotherapy and chemotherapy is markedly different from most solid tumours (see below), and they are usually curable, even if disseminated (widely spread) at the time of diagnosis.

They also differ in another very important respect – the production and secretion into the bloodstream of tumour marker substances, which are directly produced by the tumour in relation to the amount of viable malignant tissue present. The two main marker substances are AFP (alpha fetoprotein) and HCG (human chorionic gonadotrophin). These substances are made by quite specific and different cells within the malignant tissue, and some tumours produce one but not the other, though many produce both. Measurement of these markers in the blood allows pre-operative diagnosis to be made with certainty, even without biopsy, and is also of immense value in following the progress of these patients after treatment. Successful treatment should lead to complete abolition, to virtually zero levels, of both the substances. If, after a period of normality, one or other starts to rise, a relapse of the condition is almost certain, although the patient may feel completely well without any other evidence of recurrent disease at that early stage. All this would be of academic interest only, if we had no useful treatment for patients who are not cured by initial surgery, but fortunately this is not the case, since testicular germ cell tumours are among the most chemo-sensitive of all adult tumours, and the seminomas, which tend to affect a slightly older age group, are extremely responsive to radiotherapy as well.

In the first instance, however, staging and surgical removal of the primary site are the important consideration. With chest X-ray and abdominal scanning to supplement thorough clinical examination and tumour marker studies, most patients can be shown either to have localised disease (stage 1) or definite evidence of disease beyond the primary site, with various stages assigned to increasing degrees of involvement. The initial symptoms are usually a painless testicular enlargement, though pain, sometimes of a dragging or throbbing type, is occasionally a feature. Some patients have back pain as well, an ominous symptom because of the possibility of lymph node involvement in the pelvic or lower abdominal glands. When blood-borne spread takes place, it is generally to the lungs, and often picked up by a plain chest X-ray, though CT scanning of the chest is almost always performed as well, and is particularly important, of course, if the chest X-ray is apparently normal, since the CT scan is so much more sensitive. Most patients are between the ages of fifteen and thirty-five, with the teratoma group on average about a decade younger than patients with seminoma.

Treatment

When the diagnosis is more or less certain, the surgeon will almost invariably wish to proceed without delay to a removal of the whole testicle, an operation known as orchidectomy. This should always be done by the inguinal route, with the surgeon making the incision just above the groin. The two reasons for preferring this to simply opening up the scrotum are: first, the scrotum provides good protection against local extension of disease, and should not be cut; and second, so that a length of the attachment cord of the testicle can be removed as well, giving very helpful information to the pathologist as to the likelihood of spread. Scrotal incisions really are a very bad idea – hence the avoidance of biopsy as well. Very occasionally, the surgeon will discover that the enlarged testicle has another (non-malignant) cause, but, if so, he can simply put it back into the scrotum again and sew up the wound. He won't be wrong very often, though, particularly if his junior staff are well trained and pre-operative blood marker studies are routinely obtained.

If patients have stage 1 disease, they are increasingly being followed up without further treatment, particularly where the tumour is a teratoma. In the old days, additional treatment was often given, by radiotherapy or (particularly in the USA) extensive surgery with abdominal lymph node dissection, just to make sure that there were no microscopic metastases. These treatments are now performed less and less because of the excellent reliability of scanning and blood marker tests for follow-up, coupled with the predictability of tumour spread in stage 1 patients (i.e. those with apparently localised disease) in whom blood-borne dissemination would be very unusual without earlier evidence of disease re-developing in the abdominal lymph node area.

This policy of surveillance seems increasingly justified, although not all centres are agreed that it is the right way forward in seminoma, since the traditional treatment with post-operative radiotherapy has been so successful in this group, as a result of their quite remarkable sensitivity and responsiveness to radiation therapy. For this reason, only small doses of radiotherapy need be given to the abdominal and pelvic lymph node areas, generally without any long-term disadvantage. The other problem with seminomas is they don't make the tumour markers that teratomas do, so their progress is much more difficult to follow, as repeat blood tests are generally unhelpful. The dilemma persists, and many of the best centres are currently entering patients into clinical studies of one or other type of treatment. A recent interesting proposal for these seminoma patients currently under trial, is the possibility of using just a single course of single agent, post-operative chemotherapy, on the grounds that this may well be enough in patients who already have an excellent prognosis anyway. In my view, patients offered the chance of entering such studies should take the opportunity, since, in the UK, they are particularly well thought out, and the questions asked are invariably important.

Although uncommon, testicular tumours are the most important cause of cancer in men between the ages of fifteen and thirty. The overwhelming majority of patients are completely cured, either by surgery alone (most stage 1 cases) or by surgery with post-operative chemotherapy, which is likely to be given over a three- to four-month period, generally with four courses of drugs. Details do, of course, vary from centre to centre, but most large hospitals use either cisplatin or carboplatin, together with bleomycin and etoposide (see chapter 5). The drugs are generally pretty well tolerated, particularly with modern anti-nausea treatments, in marked contrast to the situation I remember in the 1970s, when chemotherapy for testicular tumours was really taking off, but invariably made patients dreadfully ill before (sometimes) curing them.

Life with only one testicle is perfectly OK. There should not be any alteration to sexual potency, since the male hormone (testosterone) from a single testicle is more than enough. Even where both testes have been involved (it does occasionally happen) and have to be removed, the male hormones can be replaced by injection, many patients requiring them approximately every two or three months. These restore the normal levels of testosterone in the majority of cases. Fertility, however, is another matter. There is a small but significant group of patients with testicular tumours who clearly are subfertile, right from the outset, even before surgery or chemotherapy. In some patients, the testicular malignancy is even diagnosed this way, the patient coming as a member of a couple to an infertility clinic and blissfully unaware of the testicular mass that is present and responsible for his producing insufficient sperm (azoospermia). Chemotherapy certainly reduces the sperm count as well, so much so that sperm storage should always be offered prior to treatment with chemotherapy. There is no doubt, however, that many patients have restoration of adequate sperm counts as time goes by after successful chemotherapy, though this may take years. It is always a great pleasure to be able to sling out the cryopreserved (frozen) sperm samples taken three or four years beforehand, in a man who is not only cured and potent but also evidently capable of fathering a child as well – in the normal way!

Despite all this good news, there is no doubt that the diagnosis and treatment of testicular tumours does produce considerable psychological stress. After all, many of these young patients are just approaching manhood, and there is probably no worse time to be told you've developed a malignant illness, let alone of the testis. Some adolescent boys, aware of a testicular mass, keep it very much to themselves for far too long because of embarrassment or fear; fortunately, they generally turn out to have a benign cause for the mass, such as a dilatation of the spermatic cord or of the blood vessels surrounding it.

As little as twenty years ago, patients with testicular teratomas which had spread up to the abdomen or chest had very little chance of cure, but the outlook has now been revolutionised by the advent of effective chemotherapy. For patients with localised (stage 1) disease, the cure rate is virtually one hundred per cent, and even in the more advanced stages, remains above ninety per cent in large specialist centres offering the best in terms of investigation, treatment and supportive care. Although often young and vulnerable, patients with testicular tumours can expect a return to a normal life – one of Britain's most celebrated patients, Bob Champion, even went on to win the Grand National a few years ago (the horse Aldaniti wasn't exactly in first-class nick either), sparking an intense interest in the disorder and helping the public towards a recognition that cancer most certainly is not an inevitable death sentence.

Case history

PAUL'S STORY

Paul, a journalist of twenty-four, was somewhat embarrassed by his swollen testicle. He'd first noticed it a month or so before, and frankly, he told me later, he didn't quite know what to do about it. You would have thought he'd have gone to see his doctor straight away, but, for some reason, it didn't occur to him that this was the sort of thing that you bothered your GP about – after all, he felt so well!

But, in the end, he did go. By this time, it was clearly getting bigger and was about twice its previous size. There had been no pain, and, in response to his doctor's questioning, he agreed to check with his mother whether there had been any history of late testicular descent when he was a child.

He went back for the second time, after a week of antibiotics, with the information the doctor had asked for: 'When I was four, I apparently had to have an operation to stitch the testicle into the scrotum.' That just about clinched it. There certainly hadn't been any reduction in testicular size with the antibiotics, and the GP arranged an urgent appointment with the local urologist. Several blood tests and a testicular ultrasound later, it was clear that this must certainly be a malignant testicular tumour – the AFP was 468 and the HCG 1,500. The testicular ultrasound had confirmed that this was a solid, not a cystic, mass.

Paul was admitted to hospital in a state of considerable anxiety. He couldn't quite believe what was happening to him, nor that the surgeon could possibly be right when he assured him that one testicle is all you need. It just didn't seem to add up. His sense of foreboding was all the stronger when the post-operative scanning tests confirmed evidence of glandular disease in the abdomen, with only a modest fall in the circulating marker levels. Histologically, this had proven to be a mixed testicular teratoma, and the oncologist was blunt: 'You certainly need chemotherapy, you need it now, and it'll almost certainly cure you.' 'I can't say I much fancy it,' said Paul. 'Unavoidable, I'm afraid,' said the oncologist, 'if you want to live, that is.' That did it. Paul agreed, and, not being one of life's more compliant individuals, later insisted that the subsequent four months were like stepping on and off a conveyor belt dragging you unwillingly along and entirely out of control.

Five years after the treatment, Paul's wife presented him with a son, and his annual follow-up visits are now more for our students' and trainees' benefit than his own. With testicular teratomas, patients who have achieved three trouble-free years from diagnosis are virtually always cured so strictly speaking, we don't need to be all that vigilant.

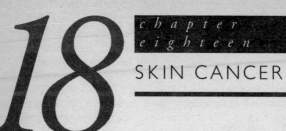

chapter eighteen

SKIN CANCER

The skin is the largest and most accessible organ in the body, subject to all sorts of potentially harmful influences, including sunlight. Perhaps we should not be surprised that skin cancers are the commonest of all malignancies. Many people are well aware of the rising incidence of some types of skin cancer, almost certainly related to our predilection for sun exposure, together with an increase in frequency of holidays in hot climates abroad, and the serious disruption of the protective ozone layer.

Causes of skin cancer

It has been known for over two centuries that skin cancers can develop as a result of directly applied carcinogens, the earliest example being the observation of Sir Percivall Pott over 200 years ago that chimney sweeps often developed a form of cancer of the scrotum because of the direct exposure to soot in the chimney flue. Other occupational skin cancers were discovered during the last century and, more recently, it has become apparent that radiation, so often used to cure cancer, can itself produce skin cancers – particularly, it seems, when given at rather low dosage. For example, it used to be common to treat ringworm of the scalp with radiation therapy, but this has now been totally discredited because of the unacceptable incidence of cancers which developed later on within the irradiated area.

As far as sunlight is concerned, there is no doubt at all of its importance in the development of skin cancers. The epidemiology of skin tumours is directly in proportion to the intensity of sunlight, so they are far more common in Australia and South Africa, for example, than in Europe. In the UK most skin cancers occur on some exposed part of the body, particularly the scalp and face. Skin cancers are far more common in pale-skinned than coloured races, particularly those with very pale, Celtic colouring.

Immune suppression is also important. Patients with transplanted kidneys or other organs, who need long-term immunosuppressive therapy, are probably a hundred times more likely to develop skin cancers, and in AIDS, one of the commonest associated conditions is Kaposi's sarcoma, generally a multi-focal type of skin malignancy and previously extremely uncommon. In addition, there are one or two inherited disorders in which skin malignancy is more prevalent, including albinism (loss of skin pigment, with an unusual and striking degree of pallor of the skin) and Gorlin's syndrome, characterised by multiple skin tumours and skeletal abnormalities.

Symptoms, diagnosis and treatment

Reducing the rapidly rising incidence of skin cancer has become a major health priority. It really is important, when sunbathing or skiing, to provide protection from burning, most particularly in childhood. Although the public are becoming increasingly aware of the dangers, it is hard to see the incidence of skin cancers falling, and education has largely shifted towards early detection of potentially dangerous skin lesions. Any pigmented or crusted area which becomes painful, or starts to blister or bleed, should be taken seriously. Far better to bother the doctor with a trivial skin lesion than to miss a potentially serious one at a stage when it is still easily dealt with. The main types of skin cancer are basal cell and squamous cell carcinoma, melanoma, Kaposi's sarcoma and skin lymphoma. The first two (basal and squamous cell carcinomas) are much the commonest, indeed the basal cell carcinoma (often known as a rodent ulcer) accounts for about three-quarters of all cases of skin malignancy in the Western world.

·BASAL CELL CARCINOMAS

These are commoner with increasing age and are unusual below the age of thirty, apart from the few cases that present as a result of an inherited disorder or early exposure to radiation. They have a very characteristic appearance and invade and destroy the skin locally, without any tendency to metastasise to other parts of the body. They are usually about 2 to 5 millimetres when diagnosed, and are typically painless, but often itchy. Usually there is a rolled 'pearly' edge, and they do not provoke any local lymph node involvement. They are particularly common on the scalp and face, especially around the eyes and nose. Occasionally, if neglected, they can grow to a very large size.

They are usually curable. Surgery and radiotherapy are equally effective, and the treatment recommendation will often depend on the preference of the dermatologist and the quality of local services. Radiotherapy has the advantage that the patient avoids an operation and loss of local tissues, though, in truth, most such operations are small and very straightforward, generally accomplished under local anaesthesia. Although radiotherapy takes longer (typically two to three weeks of treatment, though not necessarily every day) it can be preferable, for example around the eyes, where surgery may cause damage to the eyelids and possible difficulties in closure and protection of the eye. With large rodent ulcers, wider surgery and skin grafting may be the best form of treatment.

SQUAMOUS CELL CARCINOMAS

Squamous cell carcinomas of the skin are slightly more dangerous in that they do have the capacity to produce local lymphatic invasion with nodal enlargement. They also tend to spread more laterally under the skin surface, an important point when considering treatment. Like basal cell carcinomas, they are generally caused by sunlight exposure, and therefore have a similar distribution – face, scalp, neck, hands and forearms. They occasionally occur in areas of previous radiation exposure, and if so, are likely to be both clinically and pathologically more aggressive than other types, though the interval between the radiation exposure and the later development of the cancer is generally about twenty years.

Treatment by surgery or radiotherapy is generally very effective, though a wider area has to be excised (or irradiated) than in the case of basal cell carcinomas, because of the pathological characteristics of these tumours and, in particular, their greater degree of lateral (sideways) spread. Patients with lymph node involvement are generally treated by surgery, both for the primary tumour and the nodal metastases. Skin grafting may be necessary if substantial areas of skin have to be removed, but the cosmetic results are usually very good.

MALIGNANT MELANOMAS

Malignant melanoma, the commonest and most feared type of pigmented skin malignancy, is a different kettle of fish. Much more dangerous than either basal or squamous cell cancers, it has dramatically increased in incidence over the past twenty years, and is particularly common in Australia, New Zealand and South Africa, where the risk is about ten times as great as in the UK. Again, its incidence increases with age, and it chiefly occurs on sun-exposed areas, far more commonly in whites than blacks, probably as a result of the effectiveness of pigmented skin in screening out solar ultraviolet light, which is so important in the causation of the disease.

The trouble is that it can be extremely difficult to diagnose, since all of us have freckles and moles, and we don't, on the whole, pay much attention to them, particularly those on areas of our bodies that we can't easily see. It is often perfectly reasonable to keep an eye on such lesions, but skin clinics have increasingly recognised these difficulties and become far more accessible. Any change, such as crusting, bleeding, enlargement, blistering or itching, should certainly be taken seriously and shown to the family doctor. Early biopsy is much more widely available than formerly, and a good thing too.

The overwhelming majority of moles on our bodies are completely innocent, and always remain so. However, more than half of all melanotic lesions arise from pre-existing benign naevi (pigmented skin areas), though some clearly do develop at sites of previously normal skin. Naevi which change in appearance and develop an irregular edge should be viewed with suspicion, particularly if they increase in thickness, since the most reliable guide to eventual outcome is the depth of the invasion or thickness of the tumour.

If the skin biopsy does confirm a malignant melanoma, then surgical excision is the most important form of treatment. This should be undertaken by a specialist with particular experience; plastic surgeons often have a special interest in these disorders, since wide surgical excision has traditionally been recommended, and this will often require grafting, for adequate skin coverage of the defect. This type of surgery is recommended because of the wide, intradermal infiltration that may occur with melanomas, but recent reports suggest that surgery can perhaps be rather more conservative than was traditionally recommended. Malignant melanomas often spread by nodal metastases, usually into local or regional nodes (for example, tumours on the skin of the leg resulting in node involvement at the groin; tumours on the skin or arm producing lymph node involvement in the axilla), and some surgeons recommend surgery and node removal (radical node dissection) at these sites as well. The general view, however, is that this confers no survival benefit, apart from the group in whom such node metastases are already present and at the time of initial diagnosis, usually a very adverse feature indeed, but occasionally responsive to immediate surgery for removal of the glands as well as the primary site. Unfortunately, such cases are likely to be associated with the disseminated disease at more distant sites, notably lung, liver, bone, other areas of skin and even brain. Careful thought has to be given as to the best way of dealing with such problems; chemotherapy may help, but it is often very toxic and its benefits, on the whole, are short lived.

For localised lesions which have not reached a thickness of more than 1.5 millimetres, the outcome following surgical resection is, on the whole, pretty good; in fact, the thinnest group of tumours, less than 0.75 millimetres, very rarely spread beyond the primary site, and surgery is usually curative. Radiotherapy does have a role in the management of melanoma, but is generally used for controlling secondary tumours, particularly in bone or brain, where it remains the best form of treatment we have available. There are some patients, however, who relapse very late; for this group, surgery can be helpful, for example in patients with accessible solitary late brain deposits.

Although chemotherapy is not yet very effective for melanoma, there are certainly cases on record where substantial tumour shrinkage has taken place. Australian specialists, who see far more melanoma than we do, have claimed the occasional cure, even with patients who have disseminated disease, but this must be extremely unusual, to say the least. The other interesting form of potential treatment for disseminated melanoma has been the use of immunotherapy, i.e. the use of active immunisation with agents reputed to have a stimulatory effect on the immune system. Work using BCG, or even denatured melanoma cells, has undoubtedly produced local responses in patients with recurrent skin lesions or glandular disease, though most of the responses are brief. There are also reports of very occasional spontaneous regression in melanoma, or shrinkage of established disease during a pregnancy, raising the possibility of either an active immune benefit or a clinically valuable degree of hormone sensitivity; as is often the case, however, when anecdote turns into clinical trial, the overall results, from a larger number of patients, look less encouraging than we initially thought.

KAPOSI'S SARCOMAS

Kaposi's sarcoma, originally described just over a hundred years ago, was a rarity in Europe before the onset of the AIDS epidemic in the early 1980s. In Africa, however, it is a common disorder (non-AIDS related), accounting for up to ten per cent of all cancers in East Africa. The European form of Kaposi's sarcoma is clearly a disease of immunosuppression, occurring not only in AIDS patients, but also in some recipients of renal transplants. In renal transplant cases, the immune suppression (which allows the tumour to develop) can be reversed if the immune-reductive drugs are discontinued, whereas in AIDS, of course, this is not possible, since the immune suppression is the fundamental feature of the disease. In appearance, the lesions are always pigmented, often very dark, with pigmented nodules appearing on the leg or foot, and often growing rather slowly. Ulceration may occur, or the lesions may become confluent, often with a rather brawny local swelling of the affected part. In AIDS patients, the disease more often involves lymph node and other sites, notably the lining of the mouth (oral mucosa), sometimes developing with a much faster evolution than in non-AIDS-related cases.

Most Kaposi lesions respond well to radiotherapy, and a single treatment is often sufficient, though many patients will, of course, require multiple areas of treatment, notably in AIDS cases. Chemotherapy can also be useful, but patients with AIDS are at risk of so many other problems, both infectious and malignant, that lengthy survival is unusual in this setting.

Finally, many types of lymphoma (chiefly the non-Hodgkin's variety rather than Hodgkin's disease) can occur in the skin, and these are discussed in chapter 19.

In conclusion, skin cancers are common, relatively easy to spot, and, to a large extent, preventable by a sensible approach to sunlight exposure. The majority are easily curable by surgery or radiotherapy and pose little threat. On the other hand, malignant melanoma is a far more serious diagnosis and must be recognised and treated very early. Worrying pigmented lesions should always be looked at by a GP, and, if necessary, biopsied. Many skin clinics have a 'walk-in' facility for patients with pigmented lesions, so that advice can be sought quickly. For specialists in skin cancer, there are few professional activities more gratifying than the proper treatment of a malignant melanoma picked up early and almost guaranteed to be successfully eradicated.

Case histories

JAMES' AND EDWARD'S STORIES

By a curious coincidence, James and Edward, both sixty-two years of age and recently retired from the armed forces, met in the waiting room of the skin clinic just over five years ago. They had known each other well in earlier years, but had lost touch.

James was the first to be called in. He had a small, crusted lesion just behind his left ear, about a centimetre across, which had been present for three months. It wasn't pigmented or painful, but it had certainly increased in size and had bled on two or three occasions. A small biopsy was taken there and then, and a week later, the dermatologist explained that this was a squamous cell carcinoma and could be removed surgically or treated by radiotherapy. No glands were enlarged, and there was no evidence of other skin tumours. Somewhat alarmed by the prospect of surgery on his ear, James opted for radiotherapy and came along for treatment as an outpatient on ten occasions over the next month. Six months later at his follow-up visit, we noted that his tumour had healed beautifully with no scarring or residual ulceration. Three other small primaries of a very similar nature were diagnosed and treated over the following three years, all at sun-affected sites – he'd served his country for over thirty years, chiefly in India and the Far East, paying little regard to skin coverage. For two years, now, we haven't seen any sign of new tumours, and he's certainly cured of all the treated ones.

The dermatologist was much more concerned about Edward's 'little problem', as he described it. Not so little: a 2-centimetre, heavily pigmented (almost black), irregularly shaped tumour over his left thigh, clearly raised above the surrounding skin, with a slightly pale centre and a reddened flare around it. The dermatologist thought he could feel one or two glands present in the left groin; Edward's physical condition was otherwise unremarkable.

A small biopsy confirmed the fears of the dermatologist that this was a nodular malignant melanoma – quite a thick one. He didn't much like the feel of the glands in the groin either, and conveyed these fears to the surgeon, who agreed to see Edward as a matter of urgency two days after the biopsy results had come through.

The surgeon recommended wide excision of the primary tumour, with skin grafting, together with the removal of glands in the groin, making it clear to Edward that this was quite a substantial procedure requiring a week or two in hospital. Although all went well, Edward soon realised how serious his condition was when the report from the pathology lab confirmed that melanoma cells had been found in the glandular areas as well as the apparently normal skin surrounding the obvious primary site.

He healed up well, though, and had no further problems during the first nine months of follow-up, but when he came to the hospital for a routine follow-up visit, he fell as he stood up from his chair in the waiting room. Reluctantly, he admitted to having been dizzy for over a fortnight, with two additional falls. Later that day an urgent CT brain scan confirmed that he had a small but critically sited secondary deposit in the cerebellum, at the back of the brain, which was clearly a metastasis from the melanoma. Since there didn't seem to be any further deposits, and he was otherwise clear (including a chest X-ray and abdominal scan), I asked the brain surgeon to see him, and they operated the following week. Once again, the pathology lab confirmed that this was indeed a melanoma secondary, and he came back to our department for radio-therapy treatment to the brain, which was done on an out-patient basis over a two-week period.

Somewhat to our surprise, it was eighteen months or so before anything further went wrong. In the meantime, he enjoyed an excellent quality of life and travelled to California to see his grandchildren. At the end of that time, though, he appeared in our clinic, again quite obviously unwell, even though it was just a routine follow-up appointment. The complaints were of shortness of breath and increasing weakness, and a chest X-ray showed widespread secondary tumours.

Unfortunately, the whole lungs can't be irradiated in the same way as the brain – at least, not to the same clinically useful dose. He refused chemotherapy and requested transfer to the local hospice. He had considerable family and professional support, he responded to several of the palliative measures that were still possible, even though cure was clearly out of the question. He certainly perked up after a blood transfusion (he'd been clinically anaemic), and treatment with steroids by mouth and oxygen by mask 'as required' made his life a lot more bearable. He died two weeks after settling in at the hospice; his old friend James was one of the last to visit.

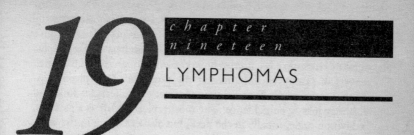

LYMPHOMAS

O ver the past thirty years or so, the outlook for patients with these diseases has improved enormously. Lymphomas are malignant disorders of the lymphatic system of the body, the glands which commonly become enlarged during infections and which are connected by a rich network of lymphatic vessels. To some extent, there is an overlap with certain varieties of leukaemia (the lymphocytic or lymphoblastic varieties), discussed further in chapter 20. Within the lymphomas, Hodgkin's disease is the most well known of the conditions, and has such particular characteristics, distinct from the other types, that the rest are generally referred to collectively (as non-Hodgkin lymphoma), though within this latter group, there are enormous variations in cell type and clinical behaviour. This group is, in fact, so diverse that there is a wide division of opinion, particularly amongst pathologists, as to how they should most logically be classified; not, I think, a topic for this chapter, but of enormous importance within the medical profession, since it is only by classifying tumours in an agreed way that we can possibly compare the treatment results from different centres.

Hodgkin's disease

Hodgkin's disease is rather a curiosity, since there is no clear agreement as to the origin of the malignant cell. Suffice to say that lymph nodes from Hodgkin's disease usually contain large cells which are the hallmark of this disorder, and thought to be the malignant component – the so-called Reed-Sternberg cell, which has very obvious characteristics under the microscope. Even though there are various sub-types of Hodgkin's disease, the lymph node usually contains large numbers of these cells. The cause of Hodgkin's is completely unknown, though there are one or two reports of family clusters, raising the possibility (completely un-proven) that there might be some type of genetic or infectious link – of course, it may just be coincidence. The most typical feature is a painless, enlarged lymph node, usually in the neck, but also occurring in the axilla (armpit) or, much less frequently, the groin area. Some patients have evidence of nodal enlargement (which they may or may not be aware of) in more than one site, and a simple chest X-ray may also show evidence of dramatic glandular enlargement in the chest, even though the patient may be completely unaware of it.

Often there are no symptoms at all, but some patients complain of night sweats, unexplained fever or weight loss, and these are extremely important since they carry prognostic weight, i.e. they affect the outcome and, if present, will almost invariably mean that chemotherapy will have to be used (see below). Other interesting symptoms include itching (often widespread) and, curiously enough, pain induced by consumption of alcohol, often, but not always, in the site of the lymph node groups involved. Although often dramatic, these symptoms are less prognos-tically important than those previously referred to. Interestingly, Hodg-kin's disease has an unusual age distribution, with one peak around the age of thirty years and a second peak in later life, possibly suggesting different causations for a younger and older age group.

The disease spreads by a fairly logical anatomical progression, generally from the initial area of nodal involvement to the next – neck to chest, for example – but not generally with a skip from, say, the neck to the abdominal lymph nodes. Conversely, patients with groin nodes are unlikely to develop chest disease without abdominal node involvement as well.

In more advanced cases, the spleen is involved, sometimes causing splenic enlargement, though there is plenty of evidence that a normal spleen in a patient with Hodgkin's disease may contain Hodgkin's tissue, and about one-third of all patients with Hodgkin's disease do have splenic involvement. Involvement of the liver, bone and lung are much less common, around five per cent overall. Staging the disease is extremely important in order to determine the degree of advance-ment. Stage 1 denotes a single lymph node site involved; stages 2 and 3 have increasing degrees of involvement (in the case of stage 3, including node groups on both sides of the diaphragm); patients with stage 4 disease have non-glandular involvement (liver, lung, bone, etc.) and are usually suffering from night sweats, weight loss or unexplained fever, often all three. About a quarter of all patients with Hodgkin's disease have these symptoms when first diagnosed though not all of these, fortunately, have stage 4 disease. Very occasionally, the nodes can become so large that they cause pressure symptoms, for instance in the chest, where the patient may have superior vena cava obstruction. Patients with Hodgkin's disease also have reduced immunity, and are more likely than the general population (or other cancer patients) to develop viral illnesses, such as shingles (herpes zoster) or cold sores on the lip and other localised herpes infections. In patients whose immunity is really poor (sometimes as a result of treatment as well as the disease itself), these infections can be extremely dangerous, even life threatening. Bacterial and fungal infections, including tuberculosis and thrush, are also more common.

TREATMENT

The clinical stage of the patient will determine the appropriate form of treatment. Apart from a routine chest X-ray, patients should also have a blood count and CT scan, firstly to identify whether there may be a degree of glandular enlargement in the chest which is not visible in the chest X-ray, and secondly, and even more important, to assess the abdomen, including the lymph node groups and also the spleen. Some years ago, there was a tremendous vogue for performing a staging laparotomy (exploratory abdominal surgery) to check whether the abdomen was involved, since there were no adequate non-invasive procedures that could do this. Nowadays, we can rely much more on radiological techniques, and very few patients require a laparotomy simply in order to decide on the correct treatment. Some centres still perform lymphangiography, a technique in which radio-opaque dye is instilled into the tiny lymphatics of the foot (first using an injection of a blue marker material in the web between the first and second toes, in order to outline the lymphatics in the first place); although this technique is elegant and produces beautiful X-ray films as the dye travels up into the abdomen, it is performed less and less, as conventional CT scanning is pretty successful and the technique of lymphangiography is so finicky.

Patients with stage 1 and 2A disease (A equals no symptoms such as night sweats, etc.) are treated by radiotherapy, and patients with more advanced disease require chemotherapy. Occasionally, in patients with stage 2B disease where the symptoms are present but very minor, a decision might be taken to use radiotherapy, without chemotherapy, particularly in patients where chemotherapy-related side effects are especially undesirable. I remember one patient, for example – a young woman from the Middle East – who was desperate to preserve fertility and happier to undergo irradiation to her neck and chest, even though she had some degree of weight loss and night sweats, than risk the long-term consequence of infertility which, for her, would have been a total disaster. Fortunately, four years later, there has been no evidence of recurrence of her disease, and we may have got away with it.

Radiotherapy techniques vary, but most radiotherapists agree that the now classic technique of 'mantle' irradiation provides an excellent chance of cure. In this approach, the assumption is made that there could possibly be microscopic spread of disease from one lymph node site to another, so in a patient with, for example, neck nodes on both sides of the neck, all the lymph node groups in the upper half of the body are irradiated in the hope that this will provide definitive treatment leading to cure. Each case must be carefully planned, since the lungs must be carefully shielded, being very sensitive to radiotherapy. We also pay particular attention to the spinal cord (which can also be damaged) and the floor of the mouth, in order to preserve normal oral lubrication. Fortunately, all lymphomas are relatively responsive to radiotherapy, so it is not necessary to go to the high doses required for carcinomas – about two-thirds of the carcinoma dose is generally adequate, with the advantage, of course, that side-effects are fewer, though the wide field of irradiation in a typical mantle treatment can pose potential problems. For patients with groin involvement, a similar logic is applied, so treatment is given to the abdominal lymph node areas and the opposite groin as well – the so-called 'inverted-Y' field.

These techniques give excellent results in the majority of patients – cure with minimal or zero side-effects. In patients with very localised Hodgkin's disease (stage 1), some radiotherapists prefer to treat the involved area of glands only, without extending the radiation field; this is a perfectly proper approach to treatment, but the patient should be aware that there is a higher risk involvement of other lymph node groups at a later stage, which will then have to be treated separately, either with more radiotherapy or, perhaps, with chemotherapy. The judgement is not an easy one, and my own view is that this form of treatment should be restricted to patients with very early Hodgkin's disease in whom the results from such treatment are really very good.

All other patients will require treatment with chemotherapy, and this, too, can be highly successful, with cure as the aim. Hodgkin's disease is generally extremely responsive to chemotherapy, and the only reason it is not used for all cases is that the side-effects, both short and long term, are generally regarded as more severe than with radiation therapy. Fertility, for example, is likely to be impaired as a result of the chemotherapy, and, just as with testicular tumours, young men with Hodgkin's disease requiring chemotherapy should be offered the chance of sperm storage. Because of the particular drugs used for Hodgkin's disease, which appear to affect sperm production in the long term, sperm storage is particularly important.

For young women with Hodgkin's disease, the danger of infertility appears rather less than with men, since the ovaries seem less susceptible to the effects of chemotherapy. Many patients continue to menstruate throughout treatment, and, if so, their chances of future fertility are excellent. In patients who stop menstruating throughout chemotherapy, there is a chance their periods will begin again afterwards (the younger the patient, the more likely this is to happen) and, if long-term infertility should develop, techniques are available at most assisted conception units to help with this. Unfortunately, it is not yet possible to preserve normal ova (eggs) from the ovaries of young women about to undergo chemotherapy – only fertilised ova or embryos can be stored in this way. I would stress, though, that the majority of young women treated with chemotherapy for Hodgkin's disease do retain fertility and should be helped towards an understanding that proper treatment of the disease, even if it does require chemotherapy, should not be compromised by anxieties about fertility; we are, after all, talking about chemotherapy with curative intent.

Most treatment programmes involve six or eight courses of intravenous chemotherapy, given every three to four weeks depending on the blood count. Some centres use one programme, some another; many of us use alternating courses of treatment, i.e. different drugs in the first and second course, and so on, in order to minimise still further the possibility of an emerging drug resistance. There is often an impressive degree of tumour shrinkage, even after the first course or two, and it is certainly possible to cure Hodgkin's disease by chemotherapy alone, though many specialists prefer to give radiotherapy as well, after the chemotherapy has finished, to the areas of previous bulk disease.

Patients with Hodgkin's disease must be carefully followed, since, if relapse occurs, further treatment is usually possible and may even be curative, even second time round. Further chemotherapy is likely to be recommended, and increasingly, in patients who are regarded as being at 'high risk', a really high-dose treatment, possibly with the patient's own bone marrow used as support (autologous bone marrow transplantation), is now being considered. This is an exciting area of research more fully discussed in chapters 5 and 8, and some patients appear to be cured by this technique even when all other avenues have failed.

Non-Hodgkin lymphoma

Non-Hodgkin lymphoma is a quite different group of disorders. The term covers a wide spectrum of diseases, all characterised by malignant transformation of lymph nodes (but not of the Hodgkin's variety or containing the Reed-Sternberg cells previously referred to). Within the group, there is tremendous heterogeneity of microscopic appearance (reflecting the varied cell types) and clinical behaviour. Although they are often symptomised by lymph node enlargement, just as Hodgkin's disease, there are many points of difference. There is no early peak in age distribution, though there is an important paediatric group of non-Hodgkin lymphoma, and a number of congenital disorders are known to predispose to lymphoma in general, of which coeliac disease (a bowel disorder characterised by abnormalities of the lining of the bowel and specific food intolerances) is the most important. Non-Hodgkin lymphoma is also far more common in patients with acquired immune suppression, for example from AIDS or renal transplant anti-rejection medication. In some types of rheumatic disorder, notably rheumatoid arthritis and Sjögren's syndrome (dry mouth and dry eyes from inadequate salivary or tear flow), the incidence of lymphoma is also increased. In Africa, Burkitt's lymphoma is a well-known disorder of young adult life which the surgeon Sir Denis Burkitt (the same one who highlighted the rarity of colon cancer in Africans and linked it to their fibrous diet) discovered and described almost forty years ago. It is of particular interest to epidemiologists and lymphoma pathologists, since it appears to be caused by a virus (the Epstein-Barr virus), which is likely to be spread by an insect carrier or vector, probably the same species of mosquito which can carry malaria.

TREATMENT

Non-Hodgkin lymphoma spreads in a more unpredictable way than Hodgkin's disease. It is much more commonly associated with non-nodal sites, notably the bone marrow, and can also, like acute leukaemia, affect the coverings of the brain (meninges), producing a lymphomatous meningitis. True, localised non-Hodgkin lymphoma is less common than localised Hodgkin's disease, and the majority of patients with non-Hodgkin lymphoma require treatment with chemotherapy. Although X-ray, blood and scanning tests will be necessary, as for Hodgkin's disease, a bone marrow test will also be required, in order to rule out involvement at this very important site. Although non-Hodgkin lymphoma can be classified in a variety of ways – cell origin, microscopic appearance (morphology), cell size, etc. – most pathologists agree that small cell lymphomas behave fundamentally differently from large cell ones, and that those which form follicular clusters, with the lymph node architecture partly preserved when viewed microscopically, also have a very different pattern of behaviour from the other group, the diffuse lymphomas.

Traditionally, lymphomas with a small cell follicular-type appearance were regarded as less serious than the large cell, diffuse variety, since the overall survival following chemotherapy was better; this view, however, has been questioned in recent years because of the effect of chemotherapy, which is different in these two types. In the so-called low-grade tumours, there seems to be no real benefit for intensive chemotherapy, and simple treatment, often with tablet chemotherapy (chlorambucil is often used), is, in the long run, as good as more intensive approaches. On the other hand, large cell diffuse lymphomas respond better to more intensive chemotherapy, and a proportion of these appear to be genuinely curable by such treatment, in contrast to the low-grade group in which, at the end of the day, very few, if any, patients are truly curable, even though lengthy survival is the rule. The question of whether we should continue to regard low-grade and high-grade non-Hodgkin's lymphoma in the same old way, despite the prospect of curing more patients with high-grade disease, has become a controversial issue. As one might expect, a number of lymphoma centres are urgently addressing the question of whether or not really high-dose treatment (again, with autologous bone marrow transplantation or peripheral blood stem cell transfusion, for example) can possibly cure more patients with low-grade lymphoma than we previously thought.

Since most patients with non-Hodgkin lymphoma have evidence of disease beyond the primary site, and often well beyond, radiotherapy plays a less important role in this disorder than in Hodgkin's disease. As well as the standard blood, X-ray and scanning tests, assessment of the bone marrow is usually required in non-Hodgkin lymphoma. Although often regarded in the past as a rather uncomfortable investigation, it's generally not too bad and quickly performed as an out-patient. The idea is to obtain a liquid sample of bone marrow cells, since these are the precursors of the circulating blood cells and give much more information than blood sampling, in several respects. Patients with non-Hodgkin lymphoma often have involvement of the marrow, yet the blood count may be normal. A simple bone marrow aspiration yields a cellular sample which can be smeared onto a microscope slide, stained and read very quickly; even more information is provided by a bone marrow biopsy, in which a core of bone is obtained, fixed and prepared like other surgical biopsy specimens in the pathology department. Obtaining a bone marrow aspirate and biopsy is simple. The chosen site is usually in the posterior part of the bony pelvis, and the area infiltrated with local anaesthetic. The bone marrow needle is then pushed in quite firmly and, generally speaking, that's that. The whole procedure should not take more than a quarter of an hour or so, and, in some ways, it's easier for the patient than having blood taken, since there's no need to search around for the vein – which can sometimes be surprisingly difficult, and extremely trying for both parties.

If all the tests are clear and the patient really does have a localised form of non-Hodgkin lymphoma, radiotherapy is often the treatment of choice, and, as with Hodgkin's disease, the dose doesn't need to be all that high. Treatment does rather depend, however, on the precise nature of the disorder. A high-grade large cell lymphoma in a young person should usually be treated with chemotherapy, even if apparently localised, since truly localised disease is highly improbable. It is well to remember that all tests have their limitations, and even the most sophisticated scanners cannot pick up a small volume of disease at a distant site.

The choice of chemotherapy in non-Hodgkin lymphoma depends largely on the cell type. Low-grade lymphomas generally respond well to simple treatment by mouth, as mentioned earlier, and the drug chlorambucil is often chosen. It is usually given intermittently for a week or two, then stopped, then restarted and so on, usually for three to six months, with careful monitoring of the patient's blood count. Sometimes steroid therapy, usually with prednisone tablets, is given as well, particularly if the disease proves stubborn and slow in coming under control. For the most part, however, patients with this type of lymphoma, who often have widespread lymph gland enlargement, respond very well. After the first few months of treatment, it is often possible to discontinue the treatment altogether, watch the patient closely and see how things go. For the most part, the lymphoma group tends to remain fully under control for months or even years, though further courses of treatment are often necessary at a later stage, as low-grade lymphomas do tend to recur. Fortunately, however, they often remain very responsive to this very simple therapy for years or even decades. Further radiotherapy is often helpful to areas of bulky lymph node involvement and is often highly effective at these sites. Resistance to simple treatment, however, does cause real difficulties, since the patient will then have to be treated more aggressively, with a less certain outcome, particularly since drug resistance often implies transformation to a more aggressive phase.

For high-grade lymphomas, intravenous combination chemotherapy is essential to bring the disease under control and to offer any prospect of cure. The disease quite often affects young patients ('young' is always a relative term, but in this context I mean below the age of fifty) and, by and large, such treatment is tolerated well, particularly with the advent of powerful, new anti-nausea drugs. The precise choice of drugs does, of course, vary, and because we cannot be absolutely certain of the best choice of agents or intensity of dose schedule, many patients are offered the opportunity of entering a clinical trial in which two or more treatments are compared. At the risk of boring you, I emphasise again that such patients are treated to the very highest standards and generally have the best possible care, assessment and outcome. Increasingly, with the advent of safer techniques for high-dose therapy, dose intensification is being studied so that we can answer once and for all the question of whether or not such treatment genuinely gives better results. For the most part, we don't yet know, and such studies are fully justified. In any event, as discussed in chapter 6, many patients are reassured and pleased at the opportunity of making a personal contribution to medical science in the area which affects them most personally.

Because of the necessity to give intensive chemotherapy in high-grade lymphomas, many of the side-effects outlined in chapter 5 will apply here. In the short term, spells in hospital, sickness, hair loss and a lowered blood count are likely to be the major problems, all, to some extent, reversible by supportive care and proper attention to detail. In the longer term, possible loss of fertility, slowly reversible peripheral nerve damage (chiefly loss of sensation) and potential cardiac weakness (from doxo-rubicin, a commonly used drug in lymphoma) are all potential threats, though, in reality, less troublesome than they might sound. As with all medical situations, the risks and potential advantages have to be balanced: when cure is the object, risks may have to be taken.

High-dose chemotherapy is more and more widely used for patients with non-Hodgkin lymphoma, particularly in patients who were initially responsive to conventional, multi-agent chemotherapy but have relapsed. A second response to the same drugs, or to second-line agents given at a conventional dose, almost always results in a less durable response than the first time round, and many centres, with the backing of the Medical Research Council and other research organisations, are currently assessing the value of higher-dose chemotherapy. This has been made possible by the advent of biological growth factors (described in chapter 8), better antibiotic support, and the techniques of autologous bone marrow transplantation or peripheral blood stem cell support (also described in chapter 8). More and more patients are now considered as suitable for this approach, and treatment results, at least from the point of view of the safety of the procedure, are improving as more centres gain experience. With peripheral blood stem cell transplantation, the potential range of applications is wide, since it is repeatable and therefore high-dose chemotherapy can, at least theoretically, be given more than once. Despite the use of these measures, however, blood counts will, of course, drop quite sharply after the high-dose chemotherapy, generally requiring a three-week stay or thereabouts in hospital before the blood recovers sufficiently for the patient to leave. The results of these studies are awaited with interest, but the general proposition, of course, is that increasing the dose intensity should lead to better and more lasting responses.

Patients with lymphoma have a relatively responsive form of cancer – responsive, that is, to radiotherapy and chemotherapy; surgery plays no part in their management, apart from biopsy at the outset and occasionally if the disease returns and there is any doubt as to the nature of the relapse. Both Hodgkin's disease and the non-Hodgkin lymphomas are potentially curable and are certainly compatible with a lengthy and virtually normal life. By and large, it is justifiable to push hard with treatment in these conditions, since there is no other way to achieve success. Even after the second or third relapse, which some patients experience, further treatment is often indicated, though obviously the greater number of relapses, the less likely a cure, and therefore the less one can justify really aggressive treatment. In Britain, we have not only the Medical Research Council, but the British National Lymphoma Investigation, who supervise multi-centre studies in lymphoma. For this and other reasons, we can claim both results and international contributions to our understanding of lymphoma which are the equal of any centres in the world.

Case history

ANNA'S STORY

Anna was twenty-seven, working in music publishing and had a promising career as a solo violinist. She and her boyfriend lived in a run-down flat and had been talking for years about getting married and starting a family – though never quite getting round to it.

As it was a particularly hot summer, she didn't pay much attention when her night sweats began, nor even when they had persisted for six weeks, to the point where she was forced to change her nightdress at least once, often twice a night. Some of the time, she felt feverish, but this, too, was dismissed. Curiously, she only became really concerned when she'd lost a stone in weight and was so exhausted when she dragged herself into work that the first two hours of each day were a complete wash-out.

Her GP found a gland in the neck and asked (perhaps rather tactlessly), 'How could you have missed a gland the size of a squash ball?' How indeed? All too easy, when viewed in retrospect, to ask these obvious questions. The truth is that we all live with situations that develop gradually – quite apart from the denial we often use as a means of avoiding the unpleasant in so many aspects of our daily lives.

It was Hodgkin's disease, oddly enough a diagnosis that still strikes a note of dread, even though it is among the more curable of tumours. In Anna's case, CT scanning and other tests showed that the disease was confined to the upper half of the body, with abnormally enlarged glands in the other side of the neck as well as the central part of the chest. Her condition was possibly curable with radiotherapy, but it was considered much more appropriate to give chemotherapy, since the typical symptoms (night sweats, fevers, weight loss) implied a more widespread disease.

For the first time in her life, Anna felt totally out of control. She had been an extremely successful music student at Cambridge, had had no trouble passing exams, finding somewhere to live, holding onto her boyfriend or getting her career moving. Suddenly she felt let down, cheated, on the receiving end of – what? All things she discovered she didn't like.

She agreed to chemotherapy of course, and in retrospect, felt that it was the threat of treatment-induced infertility which had most upset her and had clearly focused the severity of the problem in her mind.

Mortality she could cope with, but to be rendered infertile, or even the threat of such a prospect, really brought home to her the seriousness of the illness. After just two courses of chemotherapy, her symptoms had completely abated, and the glandular lump had all but disappeared. After completing the six prescribed courses of treatment, she then went on to have local radiotherapy to the chest (with a 'mantle' field of radiotherapy) and gradually got herself back to normal.

I've previously referred to the cliché of physical scars healing more rapidly than emotional ones, but in Anna's case, this has most certainly been borne out. We are now five years on, with no signs of relapse, and, in all probability, she's cured. Although her periods, which had faltered during the chemotherapy, returned to normal, she remained somewhat withdrawn and, unexpectedly, more anxious than ever about her infertility until six months ago, when her periods stopped altogether and, to her amazement (but not ours), her pregnancy test proved positive.

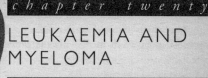

20
LEUKAEMIA AND MYELOMA

chapter twenty

The word leukaemia (literally 'white blood') strikes, if anything, a more fearsome note than the word 'cancer' – understandable, perhaps, since, for many years, until at least the mid-1950s, most forms of leukaemia where hopelessly incurable and often affected young children. But the situation has altered drastically over the past thirty years as a result of the development of powerful and selective anti-leukaemic drugs, together with their very careful assessment in several series of well-controlled clinical trials. National and international leukaemia groups, strongly supported by the Medical Research Council and other funding bodies, have often led the way in the application of the medical and statistical techniques so necessary to demonstrate that new treatments really are better than what went before.

Although leukaemia is often thought of as being synonymous with an extremely acute, rapidly developing illness in young people, the truth is more complex. All leukaemias are characterised by excess production of white cells in the blood, generally the cells on which we depend for fighting off infection and retaining full immunity; but different types of leukaemia affect different types of white cell (or, more accurately, white cell precursor, since this is essentially a disease of the bone marrow, not only the blood), and the characteristics of each type of leukaemia will vary as a result. Myeloma is also fundamentally a malignant disease of bone marrow and will also be considered in this chapter, though it is not, strictly speaking, a leukaemia. In all the leukaemias, the whole of the bone marrow is affected, and therefore a sample of any part of the marrow is representative of any other part. In myeloma (or, to be pedantic, 'multiple' myeloma), these areas arise as foci of specific sites of abnormality within marrow, hence the use of the word 'multiple'. Therefore bone marrow sampling, whilst often important as a means of assessment, is not necessarily reliable – since differing sites may vary as to their relative degree of infiltration by the disease process.

Leukaemia

Acute leukaemia is a group of illnesses characterised by sudden and often rapid development and disease evolution, whereas the chronic leukaemias are generally much more insidious, slower in onset and not necessarily requiring such urgent treatment.

Within the bone marrow is a whole host of differing red cell, white cell and platelet precursors, since the marrow is, of course, the site of manufacture of cells which will circulate within the peripheral blood. Although bone marrow is not evenly distributed throughout every bone in our bodies, it is widely present and mostly exists in liquid or semi-liquid form, which means that not only can a bone marrow sample be taken with relative ease (see chapter 19), but also that marrow can be collected for therapeutic purposes by multiple punctures (under general anaesthetic) into marrow-rich areas, aspirating substantial amounts of liquid marrow, often to a typical volume of about a litre. Bone marrow can be collected in this way for use in transplantation, either to another person, or, after processing, preservation at low temperature and storage (for months or even years), for re-infusion back into the original individual as an autologous marrow graft procedure.

Although red cell leukaemias exist, leukaemia is essentially a disease of excess white cell production and the consequences which follow. The commonest childhood leukaemia is termed acute lymphoblastic leukaemia. This term implies a disease of the lymphocytic white cell series, which is closely related to the abnormal cell in non-Hodgkin's lymphoma (see chapter 19). The leukaemic process, however, results in a far more primitive cell (the so-called 'blasts'), which are easily identifiable within the marrow, and essentially represent a highly abnormal, immature and malignant variant of what should have later developed as a normal lymphocyte. They are usually easy to detect and can be present in such large numbers that the total white cell count on an automated counting process may be five times greater, or more, than the normal white count in the peripheral circulating blood. By contrast, in chronic lymphocytic leukaemia (CLL), although the total white cell count may be grossly elevated, the malignant cell type and its degree of maturation and microscopic appearance are all far more normal than in the lymphoblastic variety – so normal, in fact, that patients often feel completely well with this form of disorder.

Not infrequently, it is without any symptoms at all, being discovered by chance when a blood count is taken for other reasons. Chronic lymphocytic leukaemias are very closely related to well-differentiated lymphoma and they are often treated similarly – indeed, neither condition necessarily needs treatment at all! This may sound odd, but chronic lymphocytic leukaemia is often a very stable condition, characterised only by obvious abnormalities in the bone marrow and blood picture, but with normal or near normal immunity and adequate levels of the circulating blood cells which we all need. About a quarter of all patients with chronic lymphocytic leukaemia have no symptoms at the time of diagnosis, even including some in whom the white cell count is really high, perhaps ten times normal.

The other two major types of leukaemia involve a quite different white cell abnormality. Acute myeloblastic leukaemia (AML) and chronic myeloid leukaemia (CML) involve cells from the myeloid series. Although these, too, are diseases of the white cell line in the marrow, the maturation and pedigree of the myeloid white cells is quite different from the lymphoid precursors. Myeloid stem (or true precursor) cells produce the specific white cells, termed granulocytes, which are given this name because they contain visible granules when stained appropriately and viewed by standard microscopic techniques, and more importantly, have a specific function in the body. Their main role is to deal with bacterial infections – pneumonia, bacterial meningitis, soft tissue and wound infections and so on. Because of the failure of development of properly mature granulocytes with normal physiology, i.e. the ability to work in the required and proper manner, patients with AML and CML are subject to very serious bacterial infections of this kind, since their immunity to these diseases is grossly inadequate. Furthermore, the abnormal myeloid precursors often crowd out the marrow to such a great degree that, in both AML and CML, the other precursors, producing red cells and platelets (the tiny particles which help the blood to clot), are greatly reduced in number, rendering the patient anaemic and/or thrombocytopenic (i.e. deficient in circulating platelets). The same is also true of (acute lymphoblastic leukaemia) ALL but rarely of CLL, though this can transform in its later stages to a far more acute process. Unlike CLL, CML is an extremely serious condition, and the term 'chronic' is something of a misnomer, since it implies a slowly evolving illness which can be dealt with using a rather 'laid-back' form of therapy. In truth, however, it is a far more aggressive and frequently fatal illness than its lymphocytic counterpart, CLL. Interestingly, CML is characterised by a particular and easily visible cellular chromosome abnormality, virtually all cases of AML possessing the so-called Philadelphia chromosome, which is, in fact, a fragment of chromosome 22, first described in 1960. In almost all (about eighty per cent) patients who have been successfully treated for chronic myeloid leukaemia, often by bone marrow transplantation from a sibling donor, this chromosome fragment disappears.

SYMPTOMS AND DIAGNOSIS

The symptoms of leukaemia do, of course, vary with the type of disease. In childhood, ALL accounts of over three-quarters of the cases, with a slight male predominance. It is not, by any means, invariably a disease of childhood, however, and is, in fact, numerically more common in adult life. It is certainly known that previous radiation exposure can give rise to leukaemia – it was one of a group of diseases recognised as more common than expected after the Japanese bomb blasts in 1945. It is also more common in children with Down's syndrome, which is, in fact, a genetic disorder with an extra chromosome, number 21, a condition previously known by the ugly epithet 'mongolism'. Symptoms occur as a result of the infiltration of the bone marrow by the diseased and functionally useless cells, so the symptoms are essentially those of anaemia, thrombocytopenia and infection due to the reduction in numbers of functionally competent circulating white cells. Typically, the history may be only of a few weeks of general ill health or malaise, occasionally with fever, sometimes with bone pain. With children who have severe thrombo-cytopenia, blotches, bruises and small red blood spots (purpura) may be visible on the skin, and bleeding from the mouth, nose or other sites may occur. Trivial knocks may cause considerable bruising. A less florid degree of symptoms may be quite difficult to distinguish from much more common childhood disorders, often viral in origin, particularly if the more spectacular symptoms, such as bleeding from the gums, happen to be absent. However, a simple blood count is all that is required in most cases to make the diagnosis (later, of course, confirmed by a bone marrow analysis). With CLL, as

214

mentioned above, the patient may have no symptoms at all, but the disease is sometimes accompanied by glandular enlargement at one or more sites, or sometimes by recurrent infections, often of a rather non-specific type, presumably relating to the reduced level of truly competent circulating white cells. The spleen, as well as the lymph nodes may also be enlarged and once again, non-specific features, such as malaise or fatigue, may well be all that the patient complains of. As the disease is very unusual below the age of forty, it can, for the most part, be dismissed as a diagnostic possibility in young people.

With the myeloid leukaemias, both AML and CML, the symptoms are often rather similar to ALL, though there are slight differences. Most patients with CML have enlargement of the spleen, and weight loss and malaise are extremely common, as well as some degree of diffuse bone tenderness. Most patients are anaemic and they often, paradoxically, have a rather elevated platelet count, suggesting that whatever is driving the abnormal white cells series may be doing the same thing to the platelet precursors as well. In other patients with CML, the platelet count is low, presumably due to crowding out of the marrow space with the abnormal proliferating myeloid precursors. CML typically evolves over a period of months or years from its initial chronic phase to a more rapid trans-formed phase, in which it is much more difficult to retain control with simple chemotherapy.

TREATMENT

Treatment of leukaemia is different for each of the four main types. In all types of acute leukaemia and CML, the immediate aim is to bring the disease under control with chemotherapy, to reduce the abnormal circulating white count, and, if possible, to obliterate the malignant cell clone within the marrow by chemotherapy. For ALL, the choice and intensity of the drugs does not generally have to be quite as powerful or severe in its effect on the patient as is the case for AML. For the most part, ALL responds quickly, often to drugs which are not especially dangerous from the point of view of serious damage (ablation) to the marrow. Steroid therapy is generally used as well as intravenous chemotherapy, since cells of the lymphocytic series are often extremely sensitive to this very safe agent. It is often possible to render the blood and bone marrow of a patient (particularly a child with the common type of ALL) virtually normal within one or two courses of chemotherapy. With AML, this is much more difficult to achieve, since more intensive chemotherapy has to be given, deliberately ablating the whole of the bone marrow, including the normal elements, with the hope and intention that the normal marrow will regenerate without the malignant clone reappearing. It may take several more courses of chemotherapy to produce the desired result in AML, with a correspondingly greater danger to the patient from each of the periods of profound bone suppression during the repeated courses of treatment. With CLL, as previously mentioned, there may be no urgency for treatment at all, and if there is, it is generally along the lines of therapy as used for well-differentiated non-Hodgkin's lymphoma (see chapter 19). For CML, relatively gentle treatment using oral chemotherapy is often employed in the first instance, if the patient is in a true chronic phase without evidence of early acceleration or transformation. A number of drugs can be used, but, in the UK, the commonest are busulfan and hydroxyurea, both quite effective, and given by mouth intermittently, for several months in most cases. Busulfan is a tricky drug to handle, since it can produce prolonged white cell suppression for many weeks after its discontinuation, so it is important not to wait until the white cell count has fallen to normal before stopping it – if this is unwisely done, the white cell count may then fall to dangerously low levels during the next few weeks.

The longer the chronic phase lasts, the better. Although the Philadelphia chromosome never disappears with simple treatment, indicating that no response to this kind of therapy is ever truly complete, the disease will not generally cause serious problems during this time. Difficulties develop when the disease begins to transform towards a more accelerated phase, at which point more intensive chemotherapy needs to be given. Since CML may well develop in patients in an older age group, the real difficulty is deciding just how intensive the treatment should be, given that the disease cannot be cured other than by bone marrow transplantation, generally from a sibling donor. Treatment of transformed CML, by conventional combination chemotherapy (as for AML) does sometimes produce remissions, but these are generally not long lasting, and a patient with transformed or accelerated CML sadly has a very poor prognosis.

The good news, however, in CML is that bone marrow transplantation has, for the first time, resulted in true complete remissions, as evidenced by the disappearance of the Philadelphia chromosome, and cures in a proportion of patients. This approach has rapidly become the treatment of choice for patients under the age of about fifty who have a matched sibling donor. As previously outlined, patients are treated with very high (ablative) doses of chemotherapy, and bone marrow from a matched related (sibling) donor is infused in shortly afterwards, the object, of course, being to destroy the whole of the malignant clone and replace it with 'foreign' bone marrow which is genetically close enough to the patient's own cells not to be rejected. These patients then live the rest of their lives with their brother's or sister's bone marrow producing their necessary marrow and blood cells, a remarkable example of biological hybridisation, since the rest of the body's cells are, of course, the patient's own. Although this is also the case with solid organ transplants, such as heart and kidney, there is no transplant, perhaps, which affects the whole of the body in quite the way that a marrow transplant does.

The technique is also used (in selected cases) in patients with AML or ALL who have relapsed or are at very high risk of relapse. Techniques are evolving all the time, but it is certainly possible to recognise particular groups of patients who are indeed at high risk of relapse and ultimately death from disease, so that allogeneic transplantation (i.e. from a different donor into the recipient, unlike autologous marrow transplantation, in which the patient's own bone marrow is employed) may be justified, despite the risks entailed. Older children or young adults (particularly males, who do slightly worse than females) who present with a very high white cell count and/or very low platelet count, may be at particularly high risk of relapse and death with conventional treatment, and therefore suitable for allogeneic bone marrow transplantation during first remission, to try and avoid a relapse ever occurring. This approach is currently under study by randomised trials in Britain and elsewhere. In AML, a disease with a worse outlook anyway, allogeneic bone marrow transplantation is seriously worth considering when a matched donor is available.

The difficulties and attendant dangers of allogeneic bone marrow transplantation are much greater than with autologous transplants. Despite the close tissue match, however, this is indeed foreign tissue (unless a genetically identical twin donor is used) and the graft would, therefore, be rejected unless suitable precautions are taken to induce a degree of immunological tolerance by deliberately producing immune suppression of the recipient (i.e. the patient), using drugs which will diminish the normal rejection mechanisms. The problem, however, is that the graft remains immunologically fully competent, and this leads to the potential dangers of 'graft versus host disease' (GVHD), in which the graft actually attacks the patient, causing all sorts of complex problems in the liver, skin, marrow and elsewhere. The sophisticated art of successful bone marrow grafting largely depends on the haematologist maintaining very tight control, with eternal vigilance in the post-transplant period and careful use of the appropriate drugs to avoid on the one hand GVHD, and on the other, rejection of the graft because of an over-powerful level of residual immune competence by the donor cells.

The first six weeks or so are quite often stormy, as a result of prolonged myeloid suppression (reduction in the bone marrow capability and cellular numbers) following the very high-dose ablative chemotherapy. Patients will obviously be restricted to hospital during this dangerous phase, and may well need treatment by intravenous antibiotics, blood and platelet transfusions and immune-suppressing drugs. The object, though, is cure; there is likely to be no alternative to this intensive form of treatment.

For children with ALL, the outlook has improved quite dramatically during the past forty years since Sidney Farber introduced the first effective anti-leukaemia drug (methotrexate) in 1948. About two-thirds of children are now curable, but, in addition to the intensive chemotherapy, they require 'consolidation' and 'maintenance' chemotherapy for a long period after initial treatment (but at a lower intensity) in order to make sure, as far as one possibly can, that the leukaemic clone has truly been abolished. They may also need a course of whole brain irradiation in order to deal with leukaemia potentially developing in the coverings (meninges) of the brain, a favoured site in leukaemia which seems not to be protected by standard chemotherapy, hence the need for the radiation therapy. Development of meningeal leukaemia is extremely difficult to eradicate and may well prove fatal in the long run, so it is far better to avoid it. Testicular irradiation is sometimes used as well (with boys at very high risk because of high white count, etc.) for similar reasons, namely that the testes can act as a 'sanctuary site' which seems to be poorly protected by the circulating leukaemia drugs.

There has been much concern about the psychological, intellectual and physical development of children who have been treated for leukaemia. For the most part they do well. There may be a possibility of a small reduction in intellect as a result, presumably, of the whole brain irradiation, though this is generally minor if present at all. Only very rarely, in an otherwise fit and cured child does it cut deeply into their quality of life. The outlook for AML may not be as good as for ALL, but many patients have been cured either by conventional chemotherapy or high-dose treatment with bone marrow transplantation. For patients with AML, irradiation of the brain is not necessary as a precautionary measure, since the disease does not seem to have the same predilection for meningeal involvement.

As far as bone marrow transplantation is concerned, there is no doubt that the closer the match, the better the results. However, a very large series of almost 500 patients undergoing bone marrow transplantation for various disorders from completely unrelated donors (all altruistically offering themselves to the United States national marrow donor programme) was published last year in the *New England Journal of Medicine*. Despite the lack of total compatibility in every detail that one has to accept with unrelated donors, the results showed quite remarkably that the probability of engraftment three months after transplantation was well over ninety percent, though almost ten per cent of these later had a secondary graft failure. As expected, GVHD really was an important problem, with about half of all surviving patients still having evidence of it a year after the transplant. However, the good news was that the rate of disease-free survival (i.e. survival without any relapse) at two years with patients who had leukaemia thought to be severe enough to require a transplant, and with relatively good risk factors, was forty per cent (in the high-risk patients, the survival risk at two years was only half this figure). There are, of course, other donor panels available as well, notably the Anthony Nolan panel, and it seems certain that now we have the available technology, the indications and applications for this type of treatment to increase as the number of panel donors with known tissue characteristics (from 'histocompatibility typing') enlarges. In the large series just mentioned, the largest number of leukaemia patients was those with either multiple relapses or failure to respond to conventional chemotherapy in the first place, making these results all the more remarkable. Almost 200 of the cases were patients with CML treated predominantly in the initial chronic phase of their illness when the chance of success was at its greatest. It is worth stressing again that the results of matched related (sibling) donor transplantation are substantially better than this, but the probability of having such a donor is, of course, rather low – about twenty-five per cent (i.e. a one in four chance) – good news for all those with large families, but clearly pointing to the need for refining still further our techniques, safety measures and donor panels for unrelated donor transplantations.

Multiple myeloma

Multiple myeloma, while bearing a superficial resemblance to leukaemia in that it is a primary malignant disorder of the bone marrow, is, in fact, a quite different disease. As mentioned previously, patients with myeloma have multiple areas of abnormality within the marrow, though parts of the marrow are entirely normal. The malignant cell is, without doubt, from the white cell series, but is an unusual, large, often pear-shaped cell, quite easy to detect under the microscope and generally termed a 'plasma cell'. As well as proliferating rapidly in the marrow of patients with myeloma, these cells are capable of directly eroding bone as they grow in their enlarging clumps, causing severe bone loss at specific sites within the skeleton – easily visible on X-rays; as a result, bone pain in myeloma can be extremely severe and widespread, and fractures are common.

SYMPTOMS AND DIAGNOSIS

Because of the crowding out of the marrow by the malignant elements, both anaemia and reduced circulation of platelets (thrombocytopenia) are common. In fact the commonest symptoms in patients with myeloma (who are particularly in the older age group, generally above forty-five years of age) are anaemia and bone pain.

As if this were not enough, myeloma is a particularly unpleasant illness in other ways as well. The malignant cells manufacture and spill out into the bloodstream a protein product known as an immunoglobulin, which is normally present in the blood, but in the case of myeloma, at a very much higher level. The type of immunoglobulin reflects the type of myeloma – there are several types, some of which leak the protein predominantly into the urine rather than the blood. Although the level of this marker product can be used as a direct indicator of the patient's progress following treatment – which, of course, can be extremely helpful – the major drawback is that, in many patients, the protein passes like all other blood products through the kidney. This can severely clog it up, causing renal (kidney) failure and producing profound protein loss within the body, since several grams of protein can be excreted in the urine each day (the normal upper limit is less than one-twentieth of a gram a day). Patients who develop renal failure early in their myeloma illness have a particularly poor outlook, and the first and most urgent step is often to reverse this process, if at all possible.

Apart from the anaemia, bone pain and the consequences of a low platelet count (essentially bleeding and bruising, but discussed more fully in chapter 20), patients with myeloma may also develop evidence of recurrent infections, some of which are severe and even life threatening. This results both from the reduction in circulating white cells (leucopenia) and the fact that the normal types of circulating immunoglobulins are, in fact, reduced – despite the single spike of a specific myeloma-related increase in immunoglobulin level of the one characteristic variety.

Typically, the other major types of circulating immunoglobulin are reduced, leading to a so-called 'immune paresis', or paralysis of the immune system. This makes it much more difficult for patients to shrug off other important infections, and they frequently develop urinary, chest and soft tissue infections which clearly relate to the blood abnormalities.

TREATMENT

Like most malignant haematological disorders of the white blood cell series, myeloma responds very well both to chemotherapy and radiotherapy. The proper treatment always involves chemotherapy, although there is dispute as to just how intensive the chemotherapy needs to be when first given. The traditional approach is to use oral melphalan, a simple alkylating agent, together with prednisone (a form of steroid therapy), to which the disease is quite sensitive; about three-quarters of all patients will respond when treated with these two agents. Over the past few years, more intensive chemotherapy regimens, have been recommended, particularly for younger patients, and we now tend to use intravenous chemotherapy, either together with, or instead of, the oral medication, on the grounds that the initial response rate, and duration of response (that all-important yardstick) are rather better. In addition, some patients with myeloma suffering from severe bone pain or fracture will require radiotherapy to those sites early on in their illness, together with (or shortly after) the chemotherapy.

Sadly, however, patients with myeloma are generally regarded as having a disease which cannot fully be cured, since the disease does return after a while, even if the initial response to chemotherapy was excellent, with improvement both of symptoms and substantial reduction (sometimes even to normal) of the specific myeloma-related rise in the circulating immunoglobulin level. It might be thought that persisting with more chemotherapy after the initial response should surely improve the outlook, but, in fact, there is no point in continuing with more and more chemotherapy when a 'plateau' has been reached, i.e. a situation in which the patient will have improved clinically, with an immunoglobulin level often substantially reduced (though not necessarily to normal) and bone marrow sampling relatively normal, with no more than the permitted maximum (a little under ten per cent) of plasma cells in the sample.

It is generally best to stop treatment at this point, and to keep a close eye on things. The conventional approach would be to see how long the remission lasts (typically it is between six months and two years) and then restart treatment, often using the same drugs as before, when the patient shows evidence of relapse, either symptomatically or on biochemical or bone marrow testing. Evidence is mounting that the use of interferon (see chapter 8) can increase the length of the initial remission. This generally involves three injections a week, usually self-administered, given indefinitely until relapse.

When patients with myeloma do relapse, they may well respond again to the previous chemotherapy, but, if not, the usual approach is to switch to more intensive chemotherapy. It can be a very fine decision, though, since many patients with myeloma are well into their seventies, and it becomes increasingly difficult to justify intensive treatment with all the potential dangers. It may be better, at least in some cases, to treat the patient palliatively, which generally means local radiotherapy to painful areas and active supportive care, including rapid treatment of infection.

In recent years, it has become increasingly apparent that myeloma is one of the most sensitive and responsive diseases to radiotherapy. Traditionally, this was restricted to local irradiation of painful sites, but, increasingly, we use radiotherapy as a 'systemic' agent, in other words rather like a drug, attempting to treat the whole body. The difficulty is that high doses of radiotherapy given to the whole body would cause fatal bone marrow suppression. Either a bone marrow transplant has to be used, or the body treated one half (either lower or upper) at a time. As far as bone marrow transplantation is concerned, the problem, until very recently, has been that few patients (remember this is predominantly a disease of the over-fifties) are fit for transplantation from a matched donor, and as far as autologous marrow transplantation is concerned, it has been very difficult to render the marrow sufficiently clear of disease, i.e. to be confident that one is not about to reinfuse a marrow contaminated by the very myeloma cells one was seeking to destroy. Half-body irradiation has, in fact, turned out to be very valuable in myeloma, since it allows the whole body to be treated, in two shots, so to speak (generally six to eight weeks apart) without the need for bone marrow reinfusion. Many patients have benefited considerably from this treatment, even when fully resistant to drug therapy, and it can generally be delivered with a simple overnight stay in hospital (or as an outpatient, particularly for the lower-half treatment) with few side-effects. It can provide a valuable, symptom-free remission period accompanied by a dramatic fall in immunoglobulin levels, lasting up to several years in the most fortunate of cases.

Also very exciting, and only recently introduced, has been the increasing use of peripheral blood stem cell transplantation as a means of supporting high-dose chemotherapy (generally with melphalan, this time given intravenously) and fractionated total-body irradiation. This has dramatically expanded the potential of this high-dose secondary therapy for relapsed myeloma, since it is technically much simpler than autologous bone marrow transplantation, requires no anaesthetic, and, from the initial experience at my own and many other centres, seems extremely safe. Theoretically, there is less risk of contamination of malignant myeloma cells, and there is, of course, no risk of GVHD or graft rejection if the patient's own marrow is used. We have been sufficiently confident at my own hospital to treat relapsed myeloma patients, for whom conventional chemotherapy no longer has anything to offer, up to their mid-sixties, if sufficiently fit. The early results are encouraging, but it would be unwise to claim more than this at the present.

With the advent of systemic irradiation, new chemotherapy drugs, interferon, autologous marrow and peripheral blood stem cell support, myeloma is among the most exciting areas of haematology work at the moment. It is an illness where details of management really do matter, and, in my view, a patient's best needs are served when looked after by an experienced team who thoroughly understand the complications of the disease and are up to date with the latest developments. Myeloma may not be curable, but we can certainly do a great deal to alleviate the patients' misfortunes, often for periods of very many years.

Case history

HARRY'S STORY

Like many architects, Harry found it quite difficult to stay employed during the recession and, at the age of forty-nine, resigned from his firm and decided to go freelance. Keeping himself busy at home was important, since the work didn't exactly come flooding in. Fitting some high bookshelves one day, he stumbled, fell and broke his arm.

To everyone's surprise, the X-ray showed, unexpectedly, that this was a pathological fracture, i.e. a fracture caused by a cancerous area, with clear radiological evidence of thinned and weakened bone. 'Yes, I have had some back pain,' said Harry. 'Quite severe, actually, going back about three months, now, and getting worse.' He looked pale, his haemoglobin was about seventy per cent of what it should have been, and a full series of X-rays of other parts of the body showed several additional areas where the bone was eroded away. This looked very much like a case of multiple myeloma, confirmed by scrapings from the fracture site, taken at the time of surgical fixation of his arm, and also by the positive bone marrow test.

He was fairly young, and the haematologist felt that he should have intensive chemotherapy with an indwelling Hickman line and intensive treatment, with a view to considering him for a bone marrow transplant if he did well enough. As with many patients with multiple myeloma, we were able to watch the progress of Harry's response to treatment by charting the immunoglobulin protein level circulating in the blood and the degree of protein spillage in the twenty-four-hour urine collections. Six months after starting treatment. Harry was pretty much back to normal, his arm healed following the surgery and radiotherapy, and with blood and urine protein levels only slightly above normal.

'Why do I have to go through a bone marrow transplant?' he asked. 'Couldn't I just take my chances, now I feel so much better?' That was a good question. But Harry had chosen to forget the dire prognosis he'd initially been given (he'd insisted on knowing the whole truth). Gently, we had to remind him again that, despite his excellent initial response, the disease cannot be cured by conventional treatment, and that we felt he'd have a better chance with a transplant.

He agreed, reluctantly, and nearly died after treatment since the high-dose chemotherapy and total body radiation following the transplant reduced his blood count to a degree that we hadn't quite bargained for. Altogether, he was in hospital for a month, requiring multiple courses of antibiotics, a dozen platelet transfusions and ten units of blood. 'The first thing I learned at medical school was *primum non nocere* (first do no harm),' said a final-year medical student during a teaching seminar when things were looking grim and Harry's life was hanging in the balance; the only answer I could give was that we can't always get it right.

Three years on, the student is now a proud young registrar and Harry is doing well. The prognosis is still uncertain, but so far it looks as though it's all been worth it. He may of course have enjoyed this lengthy remission with conventional treatment – there's no way of telling – which is precisely the sort of reason why clinical trials are so essential. For Harry, the only reminder of his illness are the three-monthly visits to our clinic, the regular, thrice-weekly interferon injections he takes and the stiff shoulder. He gets his wife to do the home carpentry.

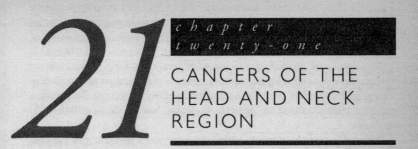

CANCERS OF THE HEAD AND NECK REGION

These tumours are, fortunately, not very common, adding up to about four per cent of all the cancers diagnosed in the UK each year. They are extremely important, though, posing exceptional problems of management and rehabilitation. They can be highly visible and sometimes disfiguring, and the treatment, particularly surgical treatment, can also lead to permanent changes of appearance.

Causes of head and neck cancer

Cancers of the larynx (voice apparatus), pharynx (throat), oral cavity (mouth, including tongue, palate, jaw, etc.) and nasal region are included in this group. Although fairly uncommon in the UK, they are much more prevalent in other parts of the world. In South China and Hong Kong, for example, tumours at the back of the nose (nasopharynx) are the commonest of all, possibly related to a diet which is high in preserved, salted fish, which might contain high concentrations of carcinogens. In parts of India, where chewing tobacco and betel nut is widely practised, tumours of the oral cavity (particularly the cheek area) are commonplace because of the direct placement of a tobacco-containing pouch against the cheek lining. In the West, though, the commonest cause of many of the head and neck tumours (notably oral cavity and parts of the throat) is a high intake of alcohol combined with heavy smoking, a situation in which the risk of developing such tumours is increased by about twenty times, in comparison with the normal population. Cancer of the larynx, a tumour clearly related to cigarette smoking, has no definite link with alcohol.

Overall, these are tumours which are commoner in men, and the past thirty years have on the whole seen a fall in incidence, probably due to improvements in dental and oral hygiene, coupled with reductions in cigarette and alcohol intake. On the other hand, there are worrying signs that, in certain parts of Europe, the number of cases (particularly of oral cancer) is starting to rise again, probably as a result of increasing alcohol consumption in some social groupings. However at other sites, notably the lip, there has been a reduction in incidence, at least in the UK, probably due to the decreasing popularity of pipe smoking, which was previously thought to be responsible for many cases of lip cancer.

Symptoms and diagnosis

Pathologically, these are typical squamous carcinomas, i.e. tumours that arise from the surface lining of the organ in question. They tend to ulcerate early, at least when situated in the mouth, so a common symptom is of a persistent, non-healing ulcer which is noticed by the patient and recognised as potentially malignant by either the family doctor or dentist. For this reason, tumours in the oral cavity are often detected relatively early, though some sites are notoriously easily missed, notably an ulcer situated in the floor of the mouth, beneath the tongue. In patients with Kaposi's sarcoma, a characteristic pigmented skin tumour often associated with AIDS, the palate is an important intra-oral site of these tumours.

In patients with cancer of the larynx, hoarseness of the voice is much the commonest symptom. Any patient going to see the family doctor with hoarseness of greater than three weeks duration should be referred to an ENT (ear, nose and throat) department for a rapid examination of the vocal cords, since early laryngeal cancer is readily detected and effectively treated. If left, however, the tumour is likely to advance to the point where cure may be impossible without laryngectomy and permanent loss of the natural speaking voice. In the pharynx, the commonest symptoms are difficulty with swallowing, since the tumour may obstruct the swallowing passage; or of nasal stuffiness and discharge, if the tumour is situated in the upper part of the pharynx, behind the nose. Surprisingly, many of these tumours are painless, though they may cause other symptoms due to their proximity to the base of the skull, and the vulnerability of the nervous pathways coursing downwards at that level.

Many head and neck cancers are associated with early invasion to the lymph glands of the neck, and it isn't at all uncommon for patients to have a swollen gland or lymph node in the neck but without any other recognisable effect or symptom. On careful inspection, a tumour might well be visibly detectable, arising from a relatively inaccessible site, such as the posterior part of the upper pharynx (nasopharynx) or tonsil. If the primary ulcer in the mouth or throat is painless, the patient may not have detected it him- or herself, even though it is clearly visible to the examining doctor. Any patient with abnormalities of this type should be very carefully examined, though the truth, of course, is that enlarged glands in the neck are overwhelmingly due to viral or other relatively minor conditions, and are either self-limiting or rapidly brought under control with a course of antibiotics.

Apart from glandular spread, head and neck tumours, as a group, do not, on the whole, disseminate to other parts of the body. Achieving permanent control of the primary site – including, of course, the neck glands – is usually tantamount to a cure. The main exception to this rule is in patients with nasopharyngeal cancers, a group which behave rather differently from all the others, with a different cell type, causation and pattern of spread. They tend to be less well differentiated than the others, with a typical pattern of early invasion of lymph nodes in the neck and a greater propensity for widespread involvement of distant sites of the body. Unlike other head and neck primary sites, radical surgery plays little or no part in their management.

Clinical staging, i.e. evaluation of the extent of tumour spread, is extremely important. Early tumours carry a much better outlook than more advanced ones, and, even more important, those where there has been no evidence of lymph node involvement do, on the whole, prove to be tumours with a relatively good prognosis (outlook); it is much more difficult to cure patients with obvious malignant lymph node infiltration in the neck. Visible and accessible tumours may be easy to stage, even without an anaesthetic, but cancers situated at deeper sites – for example, larynx and nasopharynx – will need full inspection under anaesthetic. Scanning is also important, though not necessary for every case, since it may well detect an otherwise impalpable degree of neck node involvement or give additional information as to the true extent of the primary tumour. Either or both of these features may determine the operability of the cancer.

More than any other tumour types, cancers of the head and neck remind us that cancer is not a single disease, but a group of disorders, each case bearing its own characteristics of site, local involvement, extension to lymph nodes and so on. Each of the head and neck sites requires special consideration, and although it is possible to make general recommendations about treatment, these conditions often require a degree of individualisation in the management approach. The best clinics are those where both a surgeon and a radiotherapist work closely together, seeing patients before final treatment decisions are made. It is also an area where rapid changes of management have occurred over the past ten years, with an increasing emphasis now on conservation and reconstructive surgery, to minimise, as far as possible, the damaging effects of the treatments on offer.

Treatment

LARYNGEAL CANCER

Cancer of the larynx is the commonest of the head and neck cancers encountered in the United Kingdom, far more commonly occurring in men (eighty per cent) to women (twenty per cent). It is much more prevalent in smokers, between the ages of fifty and seventy-five, and the commonest site is the vocal cord itself, rather than the other parts of the larynx, above and below the cords. Although hoarseness is by far the commonest complaint, laryngeal cancers can also cause pain or, if very large, may interfere with the swallowing mechanism. Localised tumours are confined to the free edge of the vocal cord itself, whereas more advanced ones can invade into the cartilaginous supporting structure of the larynx, paralysing the vocal cord completely. Treatment of early cases is usually successfully accomplished by means of radiotherapy; indeed, one of the greatest successes of radiation therapy is in the very high cure rate (over ninety per cent) of these tumours, without the need for any surgery whatever, generally with full restoration of the voice. The more advanced the laryngeal tumour, the harder this is to achieve, but even cases with paralysis of the vocal cord can sometimes be cured by radiotherapy, though full restoration of the voice would not occur in these patients. In Britain, where radiotherapy is widely accepted as the proper form of treatment, surgery in laryngeal cancer is often limited to the initial biopsy, for confirmation of the malignancy.

At a later stage, 'salvage' laryngectomy (removal of the larynx with permanent loss of the natural voice) may be necessary in patients if radiotherapy is unsuccessful and the tumour persists. In the USA, however, there is a greater emphasis on laryngectomy as a method of controlling and curing more advanced tumours; American surgeons seem to have less confidence in the benefits of radiotherapy, or perhaps feel more comfortable in recommending surgical resection in a wider group of patients. My own view is that loss of the natural voice is such a devastating consequence of surgery (despite the valiant attempts of speech therapists, prosthetic departments and so on) that there are very few cases where primary laryngectomy is preferable to attempting control with radiotherapy. Moreover, the use of salvage laryngectomy, in patients who clearly need it because of radiotherapy failure, can certainly result in complete cures.

Despite misgivings that surgeons sometimes express about operating on patients who have previously received radiotherapy, most patients seem to get through this type of surgery very well, despite the previous radiotherapy, so that there is little, if any, disadvantage in attempting a non-surgical cure in the first instance. Some departments recommend treatment by a combination of radiotherapy and chemother for more advanced cases, but, in my view, this is such an important issue that this form treatment should ideally be offered within a clinical trial context (see page 230).

As with many cancers, radiotherapy approaches vary considerably, and there is little to choose between a three-week course of treatment, as typically recommended at large centres in the North of England, and a six-week course of treatment, more usually recommended in London and the South. It is important, however, to be treated in a department where immobilisation shells are routinely constructed in order to keep the patient completely still throughout the treatment sessions, since precision is so important in this type of work. Moreover, there is increasing evidence to suggest that the fewer breaks in treatment, the better. It is extremely important that patients realise the importance of sticking to the recommended treatment plan, and not (as does quite often happen) waltzing off for a day or two's break here and there. That can come later. On the whole, side-effects of radiotherapy for laryngeal cancer are fairly well tolerated, though some patients do report quite troublesome discomfort in the neck area, generally short lived, or an increase in their hoarseness, before the recovery period starts. With regard to chemotherapy in laryngeal (and other head and neck) cancer, the situation at present is that it is known to improve the response rate, but, as with so many tumours being considered for chemotherapy nowadays, without any clear evidence that overall cure rates are improved.

Very few studies have been performed which might be large enough to show an overall difference, and the most impressive comes from the Christie Hospital in Manchester, where two injections of methotrexate, the antifolate drug, were given at the beginning and during the middle of a course of radical radiotherapy, with enhanced control rates in a well-matched group of over 300 patients, half of whom where treated by radiotherapy alone, the other half receiving the anti-cancer drug as well. These very promising results are currently being tested in a larger multi-centre study run by the United Kingdom Co-ordinating Committee for Cancer Research (UKCCCR), and similar studies are taking place elsewhere in Europe and the USA. The studies have to be large in view of the multiplicity of head and neck sites and the importance of gaining statistically powerful information, since the size of the benefit may only be fairly small. As with so many other sites in cancer medicine today, we need more information before recommending that the traditional, established treatment can be improved upon by the addition of new treatment methods. The hope is that chemotherapy will improve the results of radiotherapy alone, though there is no suggestion as yet that we have anti-cancer drugs powerful enough to replace radiotherapy (or surgery) altogether. Although few studies have shown an overall survival benefit with chemotherapy, a larger number have shown an improvement in 'disease-free survival', i.e. an improvement in the primary site control and an increase in the length of time between initial treatment and later relapse. This is particularly important in head and neck sites such as the larynx, since the consequences of failure are so damaging, with permanent laryngectomy or other major surgical procedures.

PHARYNGEAL CANCER

Cancers of the pharynx are a more difficult group. Cure is less commonly achieved than with cancer of the larynx, particularly in patients with cancers situated in the uppermost part (behind the nose) or lowest part of the pharynx (hypopharynx). The risk of early lymph node spread is much higher with pharyngeal than laryngeal tumours, dramatically reducing the probability of control by radiotherapy or surgery (or even the combination of both). It is generally agreed that surgery plays no part at all in the management of nasopharyngeal cancers, but the radiotherapy treatment area has to be very substantial in these cases, to cover all the potential lymph node sites on both sides of the neck. Fortunately, facial skin is so well supplied by blood vessels that the recovery from radiotherapy is very adequate, even where the original skin reaction has been severe. For tumours lower down the pharynx, surgery may have more of a part to play, though some centres rely on radiotherapy, with or without chemotherapy. For patients in this group, as well as those with oral cavity tumours (see below), the high dosage of radiotherapy necessary for cure may result in a very brisk, and sometimes painful, degree of inflammation at the back of the throat and mouth, which may be serious enough to require admission to hospital for assisted feeding by a fine-bore nasogastric tube passed through the nose directly into the stomach (in order to rest the lining of the throat). This can make treatment much easier and more effective, since it is very important that the patient does not lose weight during what can be a very tough course of treatment.

CANCER OF THE ORAL CAVITY

In the oral cavity, both surgery and radiotherapy can be highly effective. Because of the accessibility of many of these tumours, radiotherapy with radioactive implants is quite often recommended, for example with cancers of the tongue or palate, since this treatment offers a high radiation dose to the tumour itself, with a rapid fall-off in the dose to other sites. This can be used in conjunction with external beam irradiation, to boost an area of particular importance, and is often a highly satisfactory means of treatment, though limited to relatively small (less than 3-centimetre) tumours. Surgery, too, can be extremely successful, but with the potential disadvantage of loss of important areas of functional tissue. For example, even small tumours at the side or edge of the tongue are generally felt to require removal of half of the tongue (hemiglossectomy) for clearance, a fairly substantial operative procedure. On the other hand, surgical reconstruction has dramatically improved over the past twenty years, and it is now possible to recreate the lining of the mouth, the upper part of the gullet and other important sites, such that surgical resection of a primary cancer can be achieved with, in most cases, a reasonably acceptable functional result – and without the permanent dry mouth that radiotherapy can sometimes cause. The careful consideration and choice of treatment, together with a full explanation to the patient, is the kind of issue which can best be settled in a combined head-and-neck oncology clinic, case by case.

NOSE AND LIP CANCERS

Cancers of the nose and lip require a great deal of care, since disfigurement is obviously to be avoided at all costs, if at all possible. Once again, the treatment choice generally lies between surgery and radiotherapy, and there can sometimes be little to choose between them. Radiotherapy may have the edge as far as appearance and function are concerned, though for large tumours (for example those involving the whole of the lower lip), surgical resection and early reconstruction are generally preferable. What the patient needs is not only a good cosmetic appearance, but the certainty that the mouth will close properly, so that food can be chewed and swallowed without embarrassing spillage.

OTHER CONSIDERATIONS

The consequences of treatment by radiotherapy or surgery may well govern the choice of which method to recommend. With cancers of the mouth and mid-pharynx area (oropharynx), radiotherapy may certainly result in a cure, but probably at the cost of a dry mouth and some degree of oral discomfort which can be troublesome long term. There is no easy way of relieving these symptoms, but many patients manage pretty well by keeping a small bottle of water to sip throughout the day or by using an artificial saliva aerosol spray, which is now freely available. Surgical treatment, on the other hand, can lead to permanent loss of tissue which may not always be easy to reconstruct, despite many attempts at functional repair. A proper discussion of these issues before treatment is probably the best means of ensuring a satisfied patient afterwards.

When patients do have enlarged glands in the neck, it is often possible to remove them surgically using an operation which has certainly stood the test of time, the radical neck node dissection. This can often be achieved without serious, long-term consequences and with a very acceptable cosmetic result. The alternative is to irradiate the whole of the neck, and undertake such surgery only if the radiotherapy fails to control the glandular involvement. Most patients find surgery to the neck a less troublesome operation than the surgical procedure at the primary site.

Very careful follow-up is essential for all patients who have been treated for a cancer of the head-and-neck region. Most clinics recommend that patients be seen monthly during the first year of follow-up, and every two months during the second year, with gradual easing of the appointments after that. With head and neck cancers, it is usually possible to view the patient as cured if, after three years, there has been no evidence of recurrence of disease. If the cancer does recur, it is quite often possible, as described earlier, to undertake a salvage surgical procedure or, in the case of patients who have not previously received radiotherapy, offer this form of treatment. If the patient is fit and well, it is important not to give up all hope at this stage, since, as previously pointed out, head and neck cancers do not generally spread beyond the neck area. Tumour control at the primary site may result in cure, even if a second attempt, for example using surgery after radiation failure, is necessary.

As well as careful follow-up, skilled rehabilitation plays an extremely important part in management of head and neck cancers. Patients may have to learn new techniques for speech and swallowing, or may have to cope with a permanent external prosthesis if there has been surgical disfigurement to a visible part of the face, for example in the case of cancers of the nose or facial sinus areas – the cheek, for example. In the case of the patient trying to cope with a laryngectomy, many can be taught by speech therapists to produce a type of speech, with reasonable volume and intelligibility, which relies on the swallowing of air, and its expulsion up through the gullet. The resulting 'oesophageal' speech may sound a bit weird, but is often highly effective, particularly in extrovert and well-motivated people who can accompany it with theatrical gestures! One alternative, gaining increasing popularity, is the use of the speech prosthesis, which works by means of a small valve inserted into the pharynx area, and which some patients can use very effectively. Not all patients get on well with them, however, and some are more content with proper training and oesophageal speech development, together with maintaining a close link with the local speech therapy department.

For patients who have undergone operations to the pharynx, rehabilitation of swallowing is often a difficult and frustrating task. It is one thing to cure the cancer, another to provide an adequate swallowing mechanism sufficient for the patient's nutritional needs and normal social enjoyment of mealtimes. One real advantage of radiotherapy over surgery for these tumours is the lesser degree of swallowing difficulty that patients enjoy if surgery can be avoided.

As far as surgical reconstruction is concerned, there seems no limit to the ingenuity of plastic surgeons, who seem to be able to move parts of the body around more or less at will. I bow to no one in my admiration for them, but there is certainly a danger that they sometimes get rather carried away and fail to recognise that further attempts at surgical improvement may possibly do more harm than good. Once again, the best means of evaluation is by an experienced team of surgeons and radiotherapists working in close collaboration before a final treatment decision is taken.

For patients who have undergone laryngectomy, the National Association of Laryngectomee Clubs provides a wide range of booklets and other helpful advice. It can be contacted at 11 Elvaston Place, London SW7 5QG (telephone 0171 581 3023).

Other head and neck cancers

Other, rarer tumours of head and neck sites include cancers of the salivary glands, eye, orbit and thyroid. Most tumours of the salivary glands are benign and dealt with by surgery alone. Recurrences in benign salivary gland tumours are, however, often dealt with by radiotherapy as well as surgery, and you must not assume, if you are one of these patients, that the use of radiotherapy means that the tumour has 'turned malignant' even if the surgeon has reassured you that this is not the case. Under these circumstances, radiotherapy is used as a means of preventing further local recurrence.

There are, however, cases of salivary gland tumours which are genuinely malignant, and a combined approach, using surgery and radiotherapy, is generally recommended for these. Unfortunately, the facial nerve, which controls the facial muscles, runs right through the middle of the largest salivary gland (which happens to be the commonest to be affected by cancer) and permanent paralysis of the facial muscles can be a consequence either of the tumour itself, if it has eroded through the nerve, or of the treatment used to control it. New techniques are constantly being tried, to attempt a repair of the nerve and provide facial movement again, but the results of these nerve engraftment procedures are still rather poor, and plastic surgery to improve the appearance of the drooping side of the face is often all that can be recommended at present.

Tumours of the orbit, the bony structure encasing the eye, and of the eye itself, are very specialist areas where radiotherapy is generally the most valuable approach, but surgery may also be necessary.

Thyroid cancer, another highly specialist area, is a fascinating and very variable group of disorders, some of which have a remarkably high cure rate. These mostly occur in youngish women, and can be treated very effectively by surgical removal of the thyroid and, where necessary, the use of radioactive iodine. This latter treatment depends on the unique ability of the thyroid gland to take up iodine. If radioactive iodine is deliberately given, in the form of capsules swallowed by mouth, then the gland will absorb the iodine and become sufficiently radioactive that any residual cancer cells within it are destroyed by the local radioactivity; the same technique can be used for secondary deposits of thyroid cancer at other parts of the body, once the main thyroid gland has been destroyed by surgery and the first radioactive dose. This then permits a highly desirable 'self-destruct' of the secondary deposits, with the consequence that thyroid cancer is one of the few human cancers to be curable even when the tumour has spread beyond the primary site.

This general principle is unfortunately restricted only to thyroid cancers, though novel techniques are being established to try and link radioactivity, in just the same way, to tumour-specific marker substances produced by other cancers, so that in the case, say, of ovarian carcinoma, specific radioactivity with tumour targeting can be attempted. This rapidly developing sub-speciality of 'immuno-radiotherapy' is one of the more promising areas of applied cancer research being carried out at present.

Although thyroid cancers in young people are generally curable by surgery with or without radioactive iodine, the typical type of tumour in patients over the age of fifty is much more difficult to deal with, since they tend not to take up iodine (and therefore its radioactive counterpart) so readily. Nonetheless, surgical removal and external irradiation can be extremely valuable, though the overall results are far less satisfactory. For diagnosis of thyroid cancers, ultrasound of the neck, isotope uptake scans, CT scanning and biopsy of suspicious nodules are all important techniques. In the long term, almost all patients treated for cancer of the thyroid will need to take thyroid supplements in the form of thyroxine tablets for the rest of their life, in order not to develop hypothyroidism (thyroid under-activity). This is generally a very small price to pay for a highly acceptable method of treatment with an excellent prospect for cure, at least in the younger age group. In the case of a particular type of tumour known as medullary carcinoma of the thyroid, there is an important association with other tumour types, including benign overgrowth of the adrenal glands (small glands situated close to the kidney which produce adrenaline and other bioactive substances) and parathyroid enlargement (these glands sit very close to the thyroid and help control calcium metabolism). These syndromes of so-called 'multiple endocrine neoplasia' are often familial, though, curiously, it is generally only the thyroid tumour which is genuinely malignant. In patients diagnosed with medullary carcinoma, it is extremely important to screen other family members in case they are affected as well. Fortunately, this is generally achieved quite easily by means of checking their blood levels for a tumour-marker substance – calcitonin – which is usually elevated and easily detected in the bloodstream in patients who are likely to develop the tumour. Calcitonin can also be used to monitor the effect of the treatment.

Case histories

FRANK'S STORY

Frank had always been a loner. When I first met him, he was fifty-four, had had a series of building and labouring jobs, was separated from his wife, whom he hadn't seen for twenty-five years, and spent most of his evenings at the pub. He'd been on about forty cigarettes and half a dozen lagers a day since his early twenties.

His voice had been husky for two months – he had thought this was because of his smoking. Eventually, he'd turned up at casualty and they'd called the ENT registrar, who looked at the vocal cords, saw one was paralysed and realised that there was probably a tumour lurking about. A few days later, his consultant confirmed a laryngeal cancer and, jointly, we decided that radiotherapy would be the best approach, offering at least the possibility of avoiding a laryngectomy. Once again, he was treated within a clinical trial, comparing radiotherapy alone with radiotherapy plus chemotherapy: he was allocated treatment with radiotherapy alone.

He found the treatment quite tough; but although his radiation reaction settled quickly, the hoarseness did not improve, and, two months after completion of the radiotherapy, a further examination and biopsy by the ENT consultant confirmed that the tumour had not completely gone. Laryngectomy was therefore inevitable, and, realising that this was the only means of saving his life, Frank agreed.

The operation went well, and the surgeon didn't feel that the previous radiotherapy had made it more difficult. Pre-operatively, Frank received excellent counselling from the surgical team, the speech therapist who would be looking after him and from a laryngectomy patient who had gone through the same thing almost a decade before. He was in hospital for three weeks altogether, and, despite his best efforts at producing oesophageal speech by swallowing air and expelling it upwards, he never quite got the hang of it. A few months later, a speech valve was inserted in the neck and it seems to work fairly well, although it's early days.

He's come out of it all pretty well – he still gets out to the pub and the newsagent, but he isn't quite the life and soul he was before. We never did persuade him to contact his family, but he's a faithful attendee at the follow-up visits and for speech therapy sessions. He's stopped smoking altogether now, but has found it much more difficult to stop drinking, and we haven't pushed this quite as hard. His biggest frustration is not being able to make himself heard at the bar, but, as he pointed out to me a month or two back, 'I just have to get the others to buy drinks for me.'

MRS PATEL'S STORY

Originally from Bangladesh, Mrs Patel had been in England for twenty years. She'd brought up her four children almost single-handedly since her husband, Haresh, had had a severe stroke only a few years after they had arrived.

I first saw her with a note from the Department of Oral Surgery. They had confirmed her dentist's suspicions of a malignant ulcer involving the floor of the mouth and under-surface of the tongue – too extensive, they felt, for surgical removal. Her daughter was with her and, as is so often the case, acted as interpreter. She wasn't keen on conveying my thoughts too accurately, since she was anxious to protect her mother from too much bad news all at once. 'But I need to know that she realises the true position,' I said. 'Leave it to me,' she said, 'I'll make sure she understands what she needs to.'

Early during the third week of the radiotherapy, about half way through the total course, Mrs Patel developed a fierce radiation reaction. Neither she nor her daughter were keen to come into hospital, but by the fourth week, it was obvious that she would have to, in order for us to feed her properly. The family's chief concern was centred on who would run the shop. 'Maybe we could ask Daddy's friend Parviz,' said the daughter.

Fate took a hand. Parviz did well, business boomed, a dowry was found. At the six-month follow-up visit, Mrs Patel's daughter smiled shyly as she told me of the forthcoming wedding. Although Mrs Patel still complained of a painful, dry mouth, we had been able to reassure her that there was no evidence of residual cancer, and the artificial saliva spray proved quite helpful. She took it all with philosophical calm. 'Mummy says to tell you that she wouldn't have married me so well if she hadn't got ill and agreed to Parviz's coming into the shop like that.' My Bangladeshi isn't up to much, but we all beamed at each other as she left the clinic, and I made them promise they'd send me photographs.

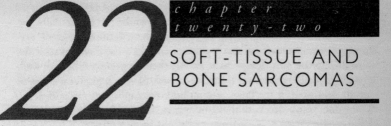

SOFT-TISSUE AND BONE SARCOMAS

S arcomas are a curious and unusual group of cancers. Unlike the much more common carcinomas, which are essentially malignant processes involving the lining (as, for example, in the bowel), covering surface (for example, the skin) or glandular structures (for example, breast, thyroid or pancreas), the sarcomas are malignant disorders of the bits in between, so to speak – the primitive 'mesenchyme', which includes muscular structures, fat, connecting tissue and bone. Not surprisingly, there is a tremendous variety of them, both of the soft-tissue variety and, pathologically quite clearly separate, the primary bone tumours – not to be confused, of course, with the secondary deposits in bone, arising from so many cancers, and very much more common that primary bone malignancies.

Causes of soft-tissue and bone sarcomas

Almost nothing is known of their cause, though a few families with a genetic disorder predisposing to sarcomas appear to have been identified. Radiation, too, can undoubtedly be the cause of these tumours, though fortunately, only very rarely. For example, there is very well-understood documentary evidence of primary bone tumours developing in the jaws of radium dial workers, mostly young women, whose job was to paint the radium onto watch faces in order to make them luminous. Little was known of the hazard of radium ingestion, and their habit was to suck the tip of their brush to a fine point to enable them to perform the task well. There are appalling cases on record as a result of very high, local doses of radium deposited in the jaws, leading both to painful erosion and decay of the bone, combined with the development of a local osteosarcoma, one of the major varieties of primary malignant bone tumour.

In a tiny minority of patients who are given therapeutic irradiation, bone, cartilaginous or soft-tissue sarcoma can develop (usually ten to twenty years later) within the irradiated area; fortunately, the risk of this occurring is well under one in 1,000, possibly ten times less than that figure.

Soft-tissue sarcomas

SYMPTOMS AND DIAGNOSIS

Typically, the patient with a soft-tissue sarcoma complains of a painless lump, most frequently on the trunk, neck, back or limb. Most lumps that people notice on their bodies are entirely benign – a bruise, perhaps (the history of trauma is often, curiously, not recalled), a lipoma, often referred to as a 'fatty lump' and of no sinister significance at all, or various types of innocent cyst or some other benign skin appendage or fluid sac (bursa), commonly occurring at or near a joint. The obviously fluid-filled ones are virtually always benign, but firm (particularly very firm) lumps should be taken seriously, and a biopsy may be necessary. As far as symptoms are concerned, that is usually more or less all there is to it, although some types of soft-tissue sarcoma are also associated with glandular involvement of the lymph node group that drains the affected area – the groin, for example, in the case of a mass on the thigh, or the axilla (armpit) in the case of many trunk or upper limb tumours. Soft-tissue sarcomas can occur at any age, and there is certainly a small peak in incidence, both for soft-tissue and bone sarcomas, around the age of twenty, after which the incidence falls again and then rises at the age of about sixty. In the soft-tissue group, there are at least half a dozen major varieties, depending on the precise type of tissue from which they originate; although I must stress that most soft-tissue lumps truly are benign, the malignant group have a great capacity for spread, chiefly by the blood-borne route, typically to lung and local-draining lymph nodes. Other important, potential sites include the liver, bone marrow and brain.

In suspicious cases, the surgeon will probably recommend surgery so that there will be no doubt as to the diagnosis; it is important for the pathologist not only to provide a description of the general nature of the illness, but also to specify which particular type of soft-tissue sarcoma it is – they all have long names and behave slightly differently from each other. The major type include leiomyosarcoma, originating from smooth muscle cells, such as the wall of the female uterus; rhabdomyosarcoma, from a striped muscle primary site, such as thigh, calf or forearm; and liposarcoma, from a fatty primary site. There are many others.

TREATMENT

If the diagnosis of soft-tissue sarcoma is confirmed, the most important treatment is adequate surgical removal, with the emphasis on wide excision and generous margins of apparently normal tissue wherever possible, and, in the case of muscular primaries, either removal of the whole organ, if feasible (as, for example, in the uterus, a relatively common primary site for leiomyosarcoma), or at least the muscular compartment from which the tumour has arisen. Surgical clearance may, therefore, have to be substantial, and, ideally, the surgeon should not encounter the tumour at all during this second, definitive operative procedure, in order to avoid spillage of tumour contents. The next and equally important part of treatment should be by means of local irradiation of the whole area to as high a dose as possible, since these tumours are not as radio-sensitive as typical carcinomas, and therefore require a higher, local dose for adequate control. This relatively con-servative method of treatment has, however, largely replaced (though not quite completely) the traditional surgical approach of limb amputation for a soft-tissue sarcoma of the extremity; in the past, this was all that could be offered.

Opinions are divided as to whether patients should then be given prophylactic (or adjuvant) chemotherapy for soft-tissue sarcomas, but, on the whole, despite many years of thorough research, this approach is not known to be beneficial, and should probably be used only within a trial setting. On the other hand, if patients do relapse at a distant site such as the lung, there is really no alternative worth considering, apart from the very few cases where relapse is late and confined to a single site which might be surgically removable (such as a single or perhaps a couple of secondary deposits in the lung). Generally speaking, it is either chemotherapy or nothing – and the chemotherapy may well be worthwhile, particularly in a young, fit patient with measurable disease which can be closely watched for response. Although a reasonable approach under the circumstances, treatment will be given without any real expectation of long-term survival or cure.

Malignant bone tumours

SYMPTOMS AND DIAGNOSIS

In the case of primary malignant bone tumours, the situation is different in several important respects. The commonest types of tumour, both chiefly tumours of adolescence and young adults, are osteosarcoma and Ewing's tumour, which, pathologically, are quite distinct from each other. Osteosarcoma is the more common and accounts for about a third of all malignant bone tumours, though their rarity is illustrated by the fact that there are fewer than 200 new cases in Britain each year. The tumour arises directly from the bone, typically in an adolescent (boys rather more commonly than girls), producing a very firm mass. The commonest site is around the knee, accounting for about two-thirds of all cases. Many give a history of trauma, but the conventional medical view is that the trauma has nothing to do with causation *per se*, but more likely brought it to medical attention. The mass itself, though always very firm, is often pain free, though not always. In the case of Ewing's tumour, the pathology under the microscope is quite dissimilar and the sites more variable, with about half of all cases occurring in the lower limb, but not necessarily clustered around the knee. It is often possible to make a fairly secure diagnosis after the X-ray, even before surgical biopsy has been performed, since the appearances of these two bone tumours are often very characteristic to an experienced bone radiologist.

In fact, it is worth saying here and now that these tumours are so rare that they should always, if at all possible, be handled by specialist panels consisting not only of clinicians (orthopaedic surgeons and non-surgical oncologists), but also pathologists and diagnostic radiologists with a particular interest in the subject. Even the site and nature of the surgical biopsy is extremely important, since getting this wrong can sometimes spell disaster or, if not quite that, then unnecessary difficulty in confirming the diagnosis.

TREATMENT

The management of these tumours should be the province of the super-specialist, and, in the UK, this is recognised by the Department of Health, which has designated two National Bone Tumour Centres, one in Birmingham and the other in London (I cannot resist the plug – my own centre at UCL participates with the Royal National Orthopaedic Hospital as the London group) with protected funding, even in these difficult days of a financially tightly controlled NHS. There have been remarkable advances in the management of primary bone tumours over the past twenty years, including the introduction of chemotherapy (now fairly standard, though new regimens are being tried out all the time, and well recognised as highly effective, particularly when given early) and the development of limb-sparing surgery.

To deal with chemotherapy first: most patients should be treated with pre-operative chemotherapy in the first instance, i.e. after surgical biopsy, but before definitive surgical removal of the primary. This not only allows a substantial degree of tumour shrinkage (and often tumour cell death) to take place, but it also gives excellent information in each individual case as to the value of chemotherapy and therefore the justification for using more drug therapy to follow on after the surgery. For both osteosarcoma and Ewing's tumours, chemotherapy reduces the risk of spread to other parts of the body (this, of course, being the most dangerous and potentially fatal complication of the illness). Radiotherapy does not generally play any part in the management of osteosarcoma, but may be useful in Ewing's tumour to mop up what cannot be achieved with chemotherapy and surgery, particularly bearing in mind that Ewing's tumour, one of a group of pathologically similar 'small, blue, round cell tumours' (not perhaps an elegant description, but an accurate one, covering a variety of pathological entities), is an extremely radio-sensitive condition. In some patients with primary Ewing's sarcoma of extremely difficult or central sites such as the central bony pelvis, radiotherapy may

243

have to be used as the primary form of local treatment without surgery, which would be too destructive to contemplate.

Limb-sparing surgery has dramatically improved the quality of life of these young patients. The concept is that the whole of the tumour area is removed, taking a generous portion of bone with it, and the whole area replaced by a tailor-made, bio-engineered metallic internal prosthesis, allowing complete preservation of the limb rather than, as in the old days, an unavoidable amputation. This is a truly remarkable feat of surgery which, particularly in the case of the lower limb generally results in an almost normal degree of functional mobility and power. The amount of work which goes into each case is phenomenal, and, in younger children with substantial growth potential, a telescopic prosthesis is sometimes used or, alternatively, a planned replacement with a longer one at a later stage. One of the trickiest parts is getting the limb length exactly right, to avoid pelvic tilting and a dissatisfied patient with an unavoidable lifelong limp. The technique is used both for osteosarcoma and Ewing's tumours, and one or two of the rarer types of bone disorder as well. Most patients require further chemotherapy in the post-operative period.

As a result of these new departures, the outlook for patients with osteosarcoma and other primary bone tumours has dramatically improved in recent years, with at least half of all patients alive and well, probably cured, at five years. Even in patients who do relapse, the use of further chemotherapy (sometimes with very intensive, high-dose regimens and autologous bone marrow transplantation) can be extremely valuable. As previously mentioned, patients with one (or even a few) pulmonary (lung) nodules at a late stage should certainly be considered for surgical removal, since this can still, occasionally, prove curative.

As the patients are generally young and subject to any number of potential long-term complications, all the points I made in chapter 19 in relation to chemotherapy for lymphomas hold good here. In addition, however, there are other problems. Some patients, notably those with a primary bone tumour situated high in the femur (thigh bone) or parts of the pelvis, will sadly need an amputation of the leg in order to gain control. Obviously this produces special problems of psychological support, follow-up and rehabilitation, too complex to go into in any real depth here. It is remarkable – and uplifting – to see how these young patients cope, and there seems no limit to what they will get up to. I have known patients with limb amputation who are far more proficient skiers than I am, who go rock climbing, sailing, and even bungee jumping. One of the real benefits of a bone tumour centre is the provision of an adolescent ward with all the noisy surroundings and incomprehensible preferences that adolescents seem to need: it really is the case that they are neither adults nor children – particularly, I think, not the latter. The right kind of nursing care, psychological support and medical input is all important. Treatment should be co-ordinated by those who really are specialists in this work, and it seems to me that the professional pains and pleasures we experience as oncologists are thrown into particularly sharp relief when dealing with this extremely vulnerable group of patients.

Case history

MATTHEW'S STORY

By the age of fifteen, Matthew was already a keen footballer and hoping for a trial with a local Premier-division junior team. After a heavy game however, he seemed to have picked up an unusually troublesome injury – a pain at the side of the knee that just wouldn't go away. Over the next month or so it got worse, and he thought there might be a swelling so eventually his mother took him to the local doctor, who arranged an X-ray.

The doctor wasn't at all happy about the report, which suggested an expansion of the lower end of the femur (thigh bone) and arranged an urgent appointment with the orthopaedic surgeon, who agreed with his radiological colleague that the changes in the X-ray were strongly suggestive of malignancy. An urgent biopsy was performed, and osteosarcoma was confirmed. Matthew was immediately referred to a well-known bone tumour unit and admitted to the adolescent oncology unit to start treatment with chemotherapy.

Throughout this time – no more than two weeks from the first visit to his GP to his admission to the teenage unit – Matthew seemed to lose all his normal reference points: school, sports, music, normal family life. It had been clear from the start that something serious might be up, and the speed of events took the whole family by surprise. His younger sister didn't much like the loss of attention, a problem that worsened considerably during the following three months.

The consultant explained that the initial treatment would be by chemotherapy followed by the removal of the affected part of bone, and replacement with an internal prosthesis (tailor-made metallic implant) in order to preserve the limb. More chemotherapy would be necessary afterwards.

The whole treatment plan went along more or less according to schedule, apart from one very severe episode of septicaemia (blood poisoning) following one of the courses of chemotherapy and the consequent sharp fall in blood count. The hair loss was manageable (he mostly wore a Yankees baseball cap – peak backwards) and the new implant was brilliant, though it was clear that movement would always be a bit restricted and he would certainly never play for Arsenal!

After that first intensive year of treatment, both Matthew and his family felt somewhat cast adrift when the chemotherapy came to an end – pleased to be shot of it, but anxious about whether his good health would continue. But as his hair returned, so did his confidence.

After two trouble-free years and pretty good marks at GCSE, he was half-way through his A-level courses, working so hard that he almost forgot to attend his routine three-monthly check. As usual, a chest X-ray was performed, but this time, the examination seemed to take longer and the professor wasn't smiling. There was a spot on the lung, possibly two. CT scanning confirmed the presence of two separate lung metastases (secondary deposits) which would have to be removed. A week later, he was admitted for surgical chest exploration (thoracotomy), going home just under a week later.

Fortunately, that was two years ago now, and no further secondaries have turned up. Matthew's at university now, reading Natural Sciences, but thinking of switching to Medicine. The family have come through fine, largely thanks to the support of their excellent GP and extended family counselling.

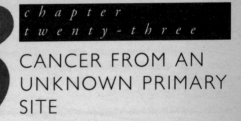

CANCER FROM AN UNKNOWN PRIMARY SITE

T hough fortunately uncommon, it does sometimes happen that a cancer which is quite clearly secondary in nature develops without conclusive evidence as to the primary site. Typical examples include lymph nodes in the neck which, on biopsy, turn out to be squamous carcinoma, or the patient with diminished appetite, weight loss and mild jaundice who is revealed, on simple ultrasound scanning, to have multiple secondary deposits in the liver, usually turning out, after a simple transcutaneous needle biopsy (through the skin) to be an adenocarcinoma. Both of these types of clinical situation occur from time to time in the complete absence of symptoms which might point the doctor towards one or other of the likely primary sites, and in every possible sense they are a real problem. To the patient, because facing cancer is always hard enough without the added burden of realising right from the outset that cure is extremely unlikely; and to the doctor, because a kind-hearted and supportive explanation of the true situation is never easy, particularly since so much weighty information may have to be given at the very first meeting. Furthermore, patients do seem to find it particularly difficult and terrifying that such a situation could arise without them detecting any symptoms – sometimes feeling as if, in some curious way, it was their own fault that they simply failed to notice.

A diagnosis of cancer is hard enough, but when the cancer appears first of all at a secondary site, it seems to make even less intellectual sense, and is therefore even more difficult than trying to come to terms with a more conventional cancer, which at least had the good manners to declare itself first of all at its initial point of departure. The doctor is in no position to say, as he or she so often can, that the management will at least proceed along the following logical lines – surgical biopsy, consideration of the best form of local treatment, etc., etc.

Symptoms and diagnosis

It is important, however, at least to make a diagnosis of what pathological type of tumour we are dealing with. A gland in the neck containing squamous carcinoma cells, for example, may well arise from a previously undetected head and neck site, such as the tonsil or floor of mouth, under the tongue. These sites may be readily apparent on expert examination, which might require a full anaesthetic to be completely thorough. If this proves to be the case, then treatment of the primary site and the neck gland is certainly well worthwhile, and may even be curative – though, as pointed out in chapter 21, patients with nodal involvement are less likely to be cured than those without it. An enlarged gland in the axilla may well prove to be an adenocarcinoma, and it is always extremely important to search most carefully for a primary within the breast on the same side, since breast cancers may be very small and undetected by the patient, yet still have the potential to produce malignant involvement at the axillary lymph node (this is discussed further in chapter 12).

Even if the specialist cannot feel a lump in the breast, it is important to request a mammogram, since this may show the typical features of primary breast cancer, and the proper management can then proceed along logical lines, though, once again, the presence of the glandular mass does confer a worse outlook. In the case of the hepatic (liver) example given earlier, there is no point pretending that the situation is anything other than extremely serious right from the outset, since liver deposits cannot, on the whole, be cured, though there are very rare exceptions, since one or two types of malignant tumour can spread to the liver, yet prove later to be strikingly responsive to chemotherapy. So it is generally worthwhile trying at least to define the pathological nature of the problem, and this means a liver biopsy, which is generally a straightforward affair, achieved by a needle biopsy under local anaesthetic.

Treatment

Treatable cancers which may sometimes appear as secondary deposits from an unknown primary site include breast, colorectal, ovary, prostate and small cell lung cancer, all briefly discussed in the appropriate chapters. In addition, there are three curable tumours which really must not be missed, since they can sometimes be treated very effectively – testicular germ cell tumours, lymphoma and thyroid cancer – again, all discussed in appropriate chapters. Even where cure is not possible, palliation, either by chemotherapy or (in the case of breast and prostate cancer) by hormone therapy, may be very worthwhile and add substantially to the patient's expectancy of life. This is particularly important in the case of patients who are likely to survive only a shortish time, and who may have much to attend to during those few precious months. In patients who have secondary deposits from an unknown primary site, the whole of the clinical, emotional and evolutionary pattern of cancer is telescoped into a much shorter time than usual, and it is important not to miss these opportunities to try and come to terms with what is likely to be a very short survival time. Perhaps the most important, strictly medical point is that it is always worth reviewing the pathology very carefully, just in case there is any question of it being a curable or potentially treatable tumour rather than a hopelessly untreatable one. Ideally, the patient will need a specialist who can offer both experience and support in this most difficult of situations.

Sometimes the patient surprises the specialist in the nicest possible way. We have certainly all seen patients who, given an almost hopeless diagnosis and a short life expectancy of a few months, have responded to treatment surprisingly well and gone on to live for two or three years. This applies both to patients who have secondary deposits from an unknown primary site and also to the much more common group of patients who develop metastases from a clearly recognised primary site. In cancer, the tempo of disease varies in the most remarkable way – so much so that it is usually unwise to be too specific about prognosis, even where metastatic disease has established itself at widely disseminated sites. These points are discussed in more detail in chapters 4, 7, 9 and 10.

Case history

JANE'S STORY

Jane was a thirty-seven-year-old opera singer who had finally begun to land some decent parts. It was annoying when her health seemed to start letting her down, just as she had found professional success. First it was one thing, then another – back pain, discomfort under the arm, fatigue, sore throat. She'd been reluctant to visit her doctor because it all seemed so likely to be work- or stress-related. But eventually, she dragged herself along, rather expecting to be told to take things easy, and slightly guilty at the prospect of wasting her doctor's time.

Unusually, it was a quiet Friday in the surgery, and there was time to talk. Her almost-retired GP, who'd seen it all and had lost his own wife to cancer, wasn't easily fobbed off. A full examination confirmed severe tenderness in the lumbar spine and an obvious mass in the left axilla (armpit), though no obvious abnormality elsewhere and, in particular, no lump to be felt in the left breast, which the doctor felt was the only puzzling part of the examination.

He did his best to explain to Jane as gently as he could that there might be something seriously amiss. Her reaction at first was one of disbelief, then dismay, then anger. It took an hour on the telephone to get hold of the surgical registrar at the local hospital, but he agreed to see her a day or two later, and a fine needle biopsy of the gland in the axilla was arranged. As expected, it confirmed an adenocarcinoma. An isotope bone scan showed a number of scattered abnormalities with a hot-spot in the lower lumbar spine, corresponding to her discomfort, and several other areas – ribs, pelvis and skull. A mammogram was done, since it seemed so likely that a cancer of the left breast would prove to be the primary cause, but unexpectedly it turned out normal.

The oncological view was that this was so likely to be a breast cancer, despite the normal mammogram and lack of an obvious primary site in either breast, that it would be totally justifiable to treat this young, fit patient as if it were indeed a breast cancer, though without the absolute certainty that this was indeed the case. Out-patient chemotherapy and radiotherapy to the lower spine were administered more or less side by side, and Jane's condition improved considerably. The mass in the axilla disappeared, excellent evidence of response to treatment.

Jane's partner was all for ignoring the illness entirely, not paying any attention to the physical or psychological traumas. He and Jane had been waiting so long for her career to take off. She, however, was more circumspect, recognising after many discussions with her oncologist that she was unlikely to survive long, and eventually deciding to preserve some of her strength and not reach for dizzy heights. 'You're making a big mistake,' said her partner.

Here's what happened: she did extraordinarily well for eighteen months, mostly pain-free, mostly off treatment and mostly securing contracts for major, but not starring, roles. At the end of that period, she quite suddenly became jaundiced, and abdominal CT scanning confirmed that there were secondaries throughout the liver and in the glands obstructing the outlets of the liver and gall bladder. The jaundice was due to build-up of bile in the skin, since it couldn't be passed in the usual way into the small bowel. As so often happens in such cases, she'd noticed that her stools were very pale and her urine had become dark.

It was possible to improve matters by passing a small tube (stent) under anaesthetic down through the throat, gullet, stomach and upper small bowel, and she also had a further course of radiotherapy, localised to the liver outlet area. She lived for a further three months. Her last outing, a few days before she died, was to Covent Garden, where a friend was singing in Janáček's *Jenufa*.

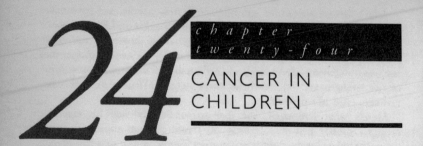

CANCER IN
CHILDREN

T here cannot be many more poignant situations in medicine – or life in peace-time – than the diagnosis of cancer in a child. It must be one of every parent's greatest nightmares, difficult to believe when it happens and well nigh impossible, for some parents at least, to take in. Yet I am determined not to reach the end of this first paragraph without saying that the outlook in children's cancers has improved immeasurably over the past twenty years, and very large numbers of children are cured. That is perhaps the most important take-away message of this whole chapter, since, tragic though it may be, the diagnosis of malignant disease in a child does generally carry with it at least.some message of hope. In particular, the two commonest types of childhood malignancy, leukaemia and brain tumour, are now much more commonly curable than ever before as a result of many advances, some dramatic, others plodding and painstaking, in all branches of paediatric oncology.

As I wrote in collaboration with Professor Robert Souhami in a medical textbook some years ago:

    🔊 *'The diagnosis of cancer in a child is an exceptional and painful test to the strength of family life. Happy families often cope better with the shock, grief and disruption. When the diagnosis has been made, the physician must take time to be alone with the parents to explain the diagnosis, prognosis and approach to investigation and treatment. About half of all children with cancer are cured; with many diseases, a cautiously optimistic account can be given. The parents will sometimes feel angry about the diagnosis and may direct this towards the doctor. Often they feel that they have been responsible in some way, in that there is a genetic factor to which they have contributed, or that the cancer has arisen as a result of avoidable physical or mental trauma or faulty diet. They need to express these feelings and must be reassured that they are not to blame.*

'Talking to children and their parents requires tact, humanity, patience and a clear head. Every new case will prove an additional test of these qualities, and the doctor will have to deal with the guilt, anguish and anger of the parents, as well as the physical and emotional suffering of the child. All children, except for the very youngest, need some account of why they are in hospital and what is likely to happen, and with older children and adolescents, these explanations will need to be accurate and complete. It is impossible to make any generalisation about how much to tell. Children of six to eight years will understand that they are ill and grasp the elements of treatment. At ten to eleven years, they will know more, and teenagers will know about cancer and leukaemia. The physician must talk to the child and try to gauge his or her feelings and understanding. For children of about eleven years or more, a personal and private relationship with the doctor is important. They often want to ask questions directly and are anxious to avoid upsetting their parents. At other times, they may feel that the truth is being filtered by their parents. The doctor should try to encourage the family to be open with each other with respect to the illness. Honesty and frankness are important in gaining the parents' trust and in helping them to participate, whereas glossing over of the facts will leave them with insufficient detail to help them understand the implications of the diagnosis and treatment.' ❧

I have included this lengthy quote, which was part of the general advice given to the profession, in the hope that it will be helpful to patients, parents and families as well. The complexity of treatment of children's tumours makes it very difficult for any doctor to provide detailed answers to all the questions which a parent or child might ask, particularly if not a specialist him- or herself in the very rarefied atmosphere of paediatric oncology. It is certainly essential that a single, experienced clinician should be seen by all to be in overall charge, though obviously, additional specialist advice may sometimes need to be sought – orthopaedic, neurosurgical and so on. This then permits that most important feature of care, the identification by both patient and parents with a single individual rather than a committee – always a danger where a large number of doctors are involved in a single child's care.

This is not primarily a book about childhood cancer, and I feel it would be unwise to attempt too much detail about the specifics of paediatric cancers. Although they are all uncommon, cancers are the commonest natural cause of death in childhood, after domestic and road accidents which sadly still come top. As previously mentioned, the commonest types are leukaemia (chiefly ALL – see chapter 20) and brain tumours. Non-Hodgkin lymphomas (discussed in chapter 19) are also relatively common, though Hodgkin's disease is very unusual. The other types common enough to merit discussion here are neuroblastoma, Wilms' tumour, retinoblastoma, and finally the paediatric sarcomas, which are in some respects slightly different from the adult diseases discussed in chapter 22.

Brain tumours

SYMPTOMS AND DIAGNOSIS

Paediatric brain tumours differ in several important respects from the adult group. The commonest single type is medulloblastoma, a developmental tumour which rarely occurs over the age of twenty-five and arises from the back of the brain, the cerebellum, with a peak age incidence of four to ten years old and a two-to-one male predominance. It forms about three per cent of all brain tumours, and the symptoms result from disturbances of the functioning of this part of the brain, together with, in a proportion of cases, raised intracranial pressure. The chief function of the cerebellum is to maintain co-ordination and balance, and specific symptoms are therefore likely to include abnormalities of gait – shuffling, falling, difficulties in walking or running, increased clumsiness; as for the symptoms of raised intracranial pressure, these include headache, vomiting and double vision. One of the most sensitive tests of cerebellar function is the heel-to-toe walking test (beloved of TV and real-life police officers though they, of course, normally perform the test for a different reason). In a child, persistent headache and vomiting, and inability to perform the heel-to-toe walking test properly should be taken seriously, though there are many other causes of cerebellar disturbance, including viral infection, etc.

TREATMENT

An urgent CT or MRI brain scan (see chapter 4) is essential and, if abnormal, a neurosurgeon (brain surgeon) will need to be consulted and the child operated on quickly. In some cases, if there is raised pressure as a result of the critical site of the tumour blocking off the normal brain fluid circulation, a draining shunt will need to be inserted into the ventricle of the brain containing the circulating cerebrospinal fluid (CSF), in order to reduce the pressure and allow the operation to proceed with safety. Various types of shunt are used, but the commonest, a fully internalised system, shunts the high-pressure brain fluid directly by means of a long tube passed all the way down under the skin of the neck and trunk, with its tip lying in the abdomen. These tubes can remain in place for many years and rarely give problems. Shunt insertion is often an essential prelude to the successful operative removal of the tumour.

Neurosurgeons have become bolder and bolder, and are now almost invariably able to remove a typical cerebellar medulloblastoma. The child is likely to be in hospital for ten days or so, and then, in the post-operative period, will need referral to a radiotherapist because surgery alone is never enough. The good news, however, is that the addition of radiotherapy as routine treatment for these children has resulted in a five-year survival rate of about sixty per cent, with most of these children cured and very few relapses beyond this point. Medulloblastoma is probably the most responsive of all brain tumours to radiotherapy, which is used not only to mop up any residual malignant cells which may have been left behind post-operatively, but also to give protective treatment to the spine.

It is important to realise that medulloblastoma, like a number of other less common childhood brain tumours, can seed down into the CSF, with secondary deposits forming throughout the spine, though not, as a rule, anywhere beyond. For this reason, a spinal MRI should always be performed in a child with this disease, though, in any event, all children (and the majority will fortunately have no evidence of spinal involvement either at the outset or at a later stage) require prophylactic radiation therapy to the whole spine. Moderate doses are used, to protect the spinal cord and nerve roots from infiltration by these deposits. If particular areas of the spinal cord are identified as abnormal at the MRI, it is sometimes possible to give them an additional boost dose, and I have certainly treated one or two children in whom there appeared to be evidence of secondary spinal deposits but, several years later, now seem cured. The traditional wisdom, though, is that children with secondary deposits in the spine are incurable and on the whole this remains true, hence the extreme priority, both in diagnosis and early treatment and just as important, routine radiation prophylaxis of the spinal cord.

This may seem like a very tall order, and the treatment does cause many problems. For a start, it takes about two months to complete, during which time children require daily treatment and have to lie very still. The skill of the radiographers and other staff treating children in special centres is phenomenal – just think about trying to persuade a fretful four-year-old to lie completely still, preferably without anaesthetic or sedation, for ten or fifteen minutes every day for eight weeks! The radiographers are the real heroes and heroines of the whole endeavour. During this period, the blood count may well fall as a result of the spinal irradiation, and a careful watch must be kept. As well as the spine and back of the brain, the whole of the front part of the brain has to be treated as well, though with a lower dose than at the back, in order to prevent seeding in this area. This means that total hair loss will always occur, though fortunately this is always reversible, and the typical thick hair of a child usually grows back pretty fast.

Some centres recommend chemotherapy as well, generally at a later stage after the radiotherapy is completed (though sometimes alongside the course of radiotherapy as well). This form of treatment is not fully established and is likely to be offered as part of a multi-centre trial of chemotherapy with the intention, as ever, to try and improve treatment results still further. This should always be discussed with the parents and child (if old enough), but these studies are, on the whole, extremely worthwhile and well run. There might be additional side-effects, though, which should be fully explained to the parents and child.

In the longer term, children treated by extensive cranio-spinal irradiation (even without chemotherapy) are likely to have a number of potential long-term side-effects. In the first instance, treatment both to the brain and spine are bound to produce a slowing down in the normal growth process. This is partly due to the direct effect on the spinal vertebrae within the path of the radiation beam, but also to the effect of the radiation on the pituitary gland (see chapter 13) lying at the base of the brain, and invariably included in the path of the radiation. Growth delay is an almost inevitable consequence of this type of radiotherapy, and can generally be detected quite quickly, by means of careful assessment in a growth clinic after treatment (in my view, an essential part of the management of any child with medulloblastoma) using fairly simple measurements and growth charts. If growth delay is confirmed, it is then possible to treat the child with injected growth hormone, and the good news is that this should restore, almost to normal, the potential loss of height. Growth hormone is now available as a fully biosynthetic substance, so there is no longer any danger of viral transmission, as was previously the case (since the growth hormone we previously used was a purified biological product).

In addition, the thyroid gland may also become underactive as a result of the direct X-ray beam passing through the spine out through the front of the neck where the thyroid gland is situated. This is generally easy to correct, if it does occur, using thyroxine replacement tablets, fortunately required only in a small minority of patients. In addition, some children will become slow to develop sexually at the time of puberty, due again either to pituitary failure or, in the case of girls, to a scattered dose of radiation directly to the ovaries, though these are usually situated sufficiently far towards the edge of the pelvis (on both sides) that the relatively narrow spinal beam misses them altogether. This, too, is generally treatable by the appropriate hormone injections or tablets when the time comes, and fertility is likely to be preserved after cranio-spinal irradiation, even if the child, now of course a young adult, needs a little bit of specialist help of one kind or another. However, these thoughts are usually far from the mind of the parents and child, aged around seven or eight and faced with a potentially fatal brain tumour.

Most of the psychological and developmental studies performed on these children, to test whether or not they are impaired intellectually by the treatment, have been reassuring. If there is an intellectual deficit as a result of this treatment to the brain, it seems, on the whole, to be relatively minor, though obviously, with more and more successes we have more and more children to study and compare with the normal age group. These are important studies, and we should know far more in ten years or so than we do now. Overall, survivors of this complex and arduous form of treatment grow up to be pretty normal, often with little or no evidence of physical or mental handicap of any kind.

Leukaemia and lymphoma

The leukaemias and non-Hodgkin lymphomas of childhood are sufficiently similar to those of adult life not to require much further discussion here. The common childhood leukaemia is acute lymphoblastic leukaemia (ALL), which is fortunately the form of acute leukaemia with the best outlook, and management of it is discussed in chapter 20. In the non-Hodgkin lymphoma group, management again follows the lines of therapy outlined for adults (see chapter 19), but it is worth mentioning that there has been an increasing emphasis on chemotherapy and a move away from radiotherapy in children, to avoid late radiation side-effects wherever possible and also in recognition of the fact that most childhood types of non-Hodgkin lymphoma are responsive to chemotherapy.

Neuroblastoma

Neuroblastoma is the next commonest of childhood tumours, over three-quarters of cases occurring below the age of four years. This is a curious tumour which arises most frequently from the adrenal gland, a paired organ situated just above the kidney and responsible both for the production of cortisone, adrenaline and other hormones. Neuroblastomas are tumours of the adrenal medulla, the part of the gland which normally manufactures adrenaline and similar bio-active compounds, though fortunately, neuroblastomas are not generally associated with high circulating levels of adrenaline.

SYMPTOMS AND DIAGNOSIS

The commonest symptom is an abdominal mass, often surprisingly large, and generally (though not always) painless. Affected children are often lethargic and irritable, and sometimes anaemic. Neuroblastomas occasionally arise at sites other than the adrenal gland, because of the embryological development of pathologically similar tissue at other sites in the body, so affected children don't always have an abdominal mass. Occasionally, lymph node (glandular) or skin deposits are the first clinical sign, or even enlargement of the liver, which is sometimes noted by a parent or more likely, by the family doctor.

The tumour can spread widely by local, lymphatic and blood-borne circulation of tumour cells, giving rise to secondary deposits in the bone marrow, liver or bone, though not generally the lungs. The diagnosis is confirmed by biopsy of an affected site (usually the primary abdominal mass), but in addition, because of the embryological derivation of the tumour cells, it is possible to pick up metabolites (break-down products) of the adrenaline-like hormones that the adrenal gland produces.

Random urine samples – or, better still, a twenty-four-hour collection – are extremely helpful, and there are at least two major metabolites of adrenaline which can be picked up in this way. A plain abdominal X-ray is also helpful, often demonstrating calcium deposits (calcification) in the primary tumour, and also in liver secondaries if present. Bone scanning should also be done since the skeleton is such a common site of secondary disease, and a bone marrow test is essential, since about forty per cent of children with neuroblastoma have marrow involvement even when the bone X-rays are normal.

TREATMENT

Treatment is by surgical removal and/or radiation therapy, together with chemotherapy in some (but not all) cases. The localised form of neuroblastoma can generally be cured with surgery alone (or with post-operative irradiation, if necessary), but children with more advanced disease will need chemotherapy as well, usually using combination chemotherapy and, in some cases, intensive treatment with bone marrow or peripheral blood stem cell support, as described in chapter 20. Unfortunately, neuroblastoma is one of the childhood disorders in which chemotherapy has made less of an impact than some of the others, since responses, though usually seen in the first instance, are of a lesser durability than with some of the other types of paediatric cancer. There is very clear evidence that the stage of disease at diagnosis (i.e. its degree of involvement within the body) gives a clear picture as to the likely outcome. Patients with localised disease are usually curable, but once the disease has spread beyond the primary site and its immediate surroundings, this is very difficult to achieve. Novel attempts at treatment, using newer drugs, more intensive approaches, bone marrow transplantation and so on, are all fully justifiable within the context of clinical trials, and parents of children treated at major centres where such trials are common should, in my view, have no qualms about discussing these issues with the oncologist in charge. Britain has an excellent record of collaborative work of this kind, with a very well-organised Children's Cancer Study Group (UKCCSG), who maintain very close links between the major centres and include some of the most outstanding paediatric cancer specialists in the world.

Following successful treatment, most children are able to live a normal life, with less in the way of potential growth failure and other endocrine abnormalities than is the case for children with medulloblastoma (described more fully on page 255). They do, however, have to be followed up carefully, since many of the drugs could have long-term consequences – likewise the radiotherapy, if used, may cause local growth problems at a later stage. A minority of patients, for example, might require treatment with a field of radiotherapy which involves approximately half of the abdominal contents on one side or the other, a particularly difficult form of radiotherapy to achieve with complete safety, since so many of the abdominal contents are extremely sensitive – kidney, liver, small bowel, etc.

Wilms' tumour

Wilms' tumour is a developmental tumour of the kidney, virtually restricted to children, with a peak age of incidence around 3–5 years and a few cases even recorded at birth. Although a little less common than neuroblastoma, it has a better outlook, even though in some cases, virtually the whole of the affected kidney is involved by the tumour process. Pathologically it has a distinct appearance, often with a mixture of more than one type of malignant cell and quite distinct from the adult varieties of renal (kidney) tumour. In about one tenth of cases of Wilms' tumour there is evidence of disease affecting both kidneys, and in a very small group, more than one family member is affected, strengthening the evidence that Wilms' tumour is a genetic disorder whose chromosome origins will shortly be unravelled.

SYMPTOMS AND DIAGNOSIS

As with neuroblastoma, the commonest feature is a symptomless, painless abdominal mass, more commonly on the left and often discovered by the parent. Sometimes the child complains of passing discoloured, cloudy or blood-stained urine; most of the other symptoms are less specific – lethargy, fever and poor appetite. Less than half of the children have evidence of secondary deposits at other sites when first examined, which is obviously good news from the point of view of curability. When the tumour does spread, it extends locally into the fat and other tissue surrounding the kidney, to local lymph node groups, and, more distantly, to the lung (unlike the typical pattern in neuroblastoma), brain and bone. The opposite kidney may also be affected as a separate secondary site.

Wilms' tumour does not produce widely recognised marker substances, but plain X-rays of the chest and abdomen will help to define the extent of the primary tumour and presence of secondary deposits, though CT scanning of the chest may also be necessary since the deposits may be too small to see on a chest X-ray. Scanning the abdomen is also important, since it will give the surgeon essential information as to the likely operability of the tumour at its primary site.

TREATMENT

As far as management is concerned, surgical removal is the most important goal of initial treatment, though chemotherapy is also highly effective, so much so that chemotherapy has even become an important part of the treatment of early cases. This, again, is in contrast to the situation in neuroblastoma – in Wilms' tumour, chemotherapy is used for virtually every case. Some centres are assessing the benefits of pre-operative chemotherapy, and the specifics of treatment will vary a little at differing centres, though generally following the guidelines issued by the UKCCSG. The position of post-operative radiotherapy is also controversial in Wilms' tumour, and currently under study. It may turn out that its traditional role, i.e. in the treatment of children with an incomplete operation (resection), with involved local lymph nodes or tumour rupture during surgery, could be at an end. Chemotherapy might potentially be more beneficial (and capable of treating more distant sites where there could also be microscopic or 'invisible' involvement) and less toxic than abdominal radiation in a growing child.

Children with Wilms' tumour generally do very well, and over three-quarters are cured. It's perfectly possible to live a fully normal life with only one kidney, of course. More difficult to cure are the bilateral cases – when both kidneys are involved – but the advent of more conservative surgical techniques and where necessary, renal transplantation, has greatly improved the outlook even for these difficult cases.

Rhabdomyosarcoma

The primary bone tumours of childhood are treated just as those of the older age groups (see chapter 22), but there is one childhood sarcoma worthy of more explanation here. This is the rhabdomyosarcoma, a tumour chiefly occurring in children between two and five years of age and with different microscopic features from the typical adult type.

SYMPTOMS AND DIAGNOSIS

In young children, the commonest variety is the embryonal rhabdomyosarcoma, which generally appears as a painless mass at a variety of sites including trunk, limb and head and neck, and the orbit, a site at which protuberance of the eye itself will be the main clinical feature. These tumours are capable of spreading widely, both to lymph nodes and also to more distant sites, especially the lung and bone marrow.

TREATMENT

As with all paediatric tumours, current management guidelines are complicated and very dependent on tumour stage, which in turn will be determined by the usual blood, X-ray and scanning tests. Progress in the management of this tumour has also been very rapid over the past twenty years. Chemotherapy is highly effective and is now given pre-operatively, after biopsy confirmation, with relatively conservative surgical resection, post-operative irradiation and chemotherapy within strict UKCCSG or other collaborative trial group protocols. In some cases, particularly the deeply situated tumours in the facial area, surgery isn't generally performed at all, in order to avoid unnecessary mutilation. Local irradiation and early (adjuvant) chemotherapy can be extremely successful, often achieving a cure with less in the way of long-term damage than if surgery were used as well.

Although several of the chemotherapy drugs are known to be valuable in this disease, new agents and more intensive dose schedules are currently under investigation, particularly for patients with secondary spread, since these of course are so much more difficult to cure by conventional means. Nonetheless, the majority of children with rhabdomyosarcoma are cured, in sharp distinction to the situation in the 1960s. In patients with local disease, the cure rate is over eighty per cent, with evidence that the survival for younger children (under the age of about seven) is better than in the older age group, though this may also relate to the stage of development of the disease when diagnosed, which remains the overriding factor from the point of view of the long-term outlook.

Retinoblastoma

Finally, retinoblastoma, which is a unique and often familial malignant tumour of the eye. The disease arises often at more than one site within the eye, from the retinal layer, that is to say the pigmented, light-sensitive part at the back of the eye. Typically the tumour spreads forward into the semi-solid gelatinous part of the eye, the vitreous humour, sometimes producing retinal detachment. The retina is the innermost layer of the eye, and extension backwards to the coating (the sclera) or optic nerve is unusual. Spread can occur either to the CSF or blood, sometimes producing secondary deposits in bone marrow, liver, lungs and other sites.

Retinoblastomas are rare, but they are particularly important biologically, and with a genetically determined familial incidence. The rate appears to have doubled over the past forty years, and this tumour now accounts for about three per cent of all childhood cancers. The increasing incidence is doubtless due to the fact that it is an inherited type of malignancy in which survival is on the increase, which then in turn leads to an increase of the number of children born to previously affected survivors, now parents themselves. The genetic transmission of retinoblastoma is both important and complex. Despite the well-recognised family clustering, most cases of retinoblastoma are, in fact, sporadic (i.e. non-familial). When inherited, the genetic transmission is via a non-sexual (autosomal) dominant gene, which means that offspring of the survivors of the hereditary form (or, as it turns out, of sporadic cases where both eyes are affected) will have a fifty per cent chance of developing the tumour themselves, since the term 'dominant' means that only one gene (of a pair) is necessary for the disease to become manifest – unlike the 'recessive' genetic illnesses in which both genes have to be faulty.

Non-familial cases are generally one sided (unilateral), with only a small risk (about seven to ten per cent) that the children of survivors will themselves be affected. Unaffected parents of a child who develops unilateral disease have a very small risk (under five per cent) of having another affected child, but in the occasional sporadic bilateral case (i.e. affecting both eyes), there is a fifty per cent chance that when they grow up, any children could then develop the disease. A further important point is that in family cases, most of the affected children will unfortunately develop bilateral disease, so that, in an apparently unilateral case, very close watch must be kept on the opposite (contralateral) eye.

SYMPTOMS AND DIAGNOSIS

Most children affected by retinoblastoma develop the disease before the age of two years, generally with a white pupil which can be quite noticeable and is sometimes picked up as an obvious difference between the two eyes (lack of the 'red eye' effect) when family photographs are taken indoors with a flash camera. The difference, of course, is due to the inability of the affected eye to reflect light in the usual way, and the white pupil is sometimes termed a 'cat's eye reflex'. Later on, children with retinoblastoma often develop a squint, increased pressure in the eye (glaucoma) or difficulties with visual fixation (for example, with reading) or with vision generally. Total blindness is not of course a typical feature, unless both eyes are grossly affected.

Early examination by the family doctor and referral to an ophthal-mologist (eye specialist) usually results in rapid diagnosis, though obviously, other diseases of the eye may be the cause of these worrying symptoms. Once again, tumour staging gives an excellent guide as to the likely outcome, and for retinoblastoma, the stage depends on the number, position and size of the tumours within the eye, features which are greatly facilitated by intra-ocular photographic techniques for permanent recording of the findings before and after treatment.

TREATMENT

As far as treatment is concerned, it has become more and more possible to preserve the eye by use of radiotherapy, chemotherapy, photocoagulation or cryosurgery (local freezing) rather than removal of the affected eye itself. The radiotherapy techniques include not only external irradiation, but a highly sophisticated form of brachytherapy (see chapter 5) in which radioactive cobalt plaques are often used, placed as closely as possible against the tumour site. With single tumours above about 10 millimetres in size, external irradiation of the whole eye is often the treatment of choice and is often achievable with adequate preservation of vision, since the retina from which the tumour arises is much more tolerant of a high radiation dose than the lens and cornea at the front of the eye. This can usually be specifically shielded without dangerously undertreating the important area. For all these reasons, treatment of retinoblastoma is a highly specialised field of oncology.

With more advanced cases, the child is increasingly likely to lose the eye, but even with bilateral cases, very good preservation of vision is often achieved. Fortunately, most retinoblastomas are sufficiently sensitive to radiotherapy for only modest doses to be required, either of external beam or brachytherapy. If the irradiation beam does have to pass through the lens, cataract formation may well occur at a later stage, clouding the vision but fortunately easily reversible by lens extraction where necessary. One important, potential, long-term complication which is more troublesome however, is the radiation-induced second tumour, particularly common in retinoblastoma and occurring in up to ten per cent of children (most frequently in those who require repeated courses of radiotherapy to control recurrent or multiple tumours). This relatively high risk of second tumours reflects not only the dangers of radiotherapy, which for the most part are relatively minor but also, for reasons which are not yet fully understood, a particular genetic predisposition to second cancers in patients with this disease.

The results of treatment are extremely good, particularly in early cases where the cure rate (with normal or near-normal visual preservation) should be virtually one hundred per cent. Thankfully, it is nowadays unusual to have to remove the eye surgically, and cure rates of seventy-five per cent are regularly achieved, even in the more advanced stages of disease. A few children, successfully treated, will later die from a second radiation-induced tumour (usually an osteosarcoma), a particular tragedy where the original cancer had been unequivocally cured.

For patients with high-risk tumours (i.e. those in whom cure is less certain), including those which have extended beyond the eye itself by the time of diagnosis, cancer chemotherapy has been used, either with single agents or drug combinations, with partial success. The precise indications for chemotherapy in retinoblastoma are not yet entirely clear, but it is increasingly used in the more adverse, locally advanced cases.

Conclusion

For many childhood cancers, the disease is rapidly brought under control, the child feels and looks well, and the clinical picture becomes more dominated by treatment side-effects than the initial damage wrought by the tumour itself. As the acute anxiety about the initial diagnosis fades in response to treatment success, so the nausea, vomiting, hair loss and disruption of school and family life all place a great strain on the child and, indeed, the rest of the family too. Siblings may feel 'left out' because of all the attention necessarily focused on the young patient, and they may also, of course, have fears of their own which they are afraid to express. In the long term, the more prolonged side-effects of treatment may produce many new problems, some previously referred to, such as intellectual and neurological impairment, growth defects, infertility and other hormone effects. Secondary treatment, if necessary, is likely to bring up all the old anxieties, and most parents and children will recognise that the situation is still more difficult than it was before, since the initial treatment had proved insufficient. Again, I will quote from the medical textbook which Professor Souhami and I published in 1994, since I think it is relevant here:

> *'Parents may be angry that relapse has occurred, and might feel that they have been wrong to allow aggressive treatment with its attendant side-effects and all to no avail. This anger may be directed at the medical and nursing staff. Even at this difficult stage, gentle explanations remain important, and the clinician in charge of the child will also need to remember that less-experienced staff may themselves need to be reassured and supported. It is important for parents to know that freedom from pain and discomfort is usually possible, and that the child's survival will not be uselessly prolonged.'*

Fortunately, many childhood cancers can now be cured, the result of a remarkable sequence of research discoveries and collaboration, both at laboratory and clinical level. In fact, studies of childhood cancer are often regarded as models to help in our attempts at defining the most promising lines of study in adult patients as well. With the advent of safer methods of supportive care, more intensive chemotherapy, and the recognition that most of the commoner paediatric malignancies are to some extent chemo-sensitive, there is every reason to hope that survival figures will continue to improve over the next decade.

Case history

PAUL'S STORY

Paul was one of those active nine-year-olds who could never sit still. Skateboarding, mountain biking, sponsored swims – he'd embraced them all with equal enthusiasm. But he seemed to be developing an odd kind of clumsiness, a tendency to fall, which eventually became quite exasperating. On the first visit, the doctor couldn't find anything specifically wrong, but a month later, when Paul had had two more falls in the street playing after school, his mother took him back and insisted on a more thorough examination. When the doctor asked Paul to walk heel-to-toe in a straight line, it was clear that the task was quite beyond him, and an urgent referral to the local paediatrician was followed within a day or two by a brain scan.

It was quite a large tumour, bang in the midline, almost 3 centimetres across. Clearly it was a case for the specialist paediatric neurosurgeon; fortunately he seemed pretty confident that it could be removed without too much trouble.

It turned out to be a medulloblastoma, the commonest of the childhood brain tumours arising in that part of the brain. The brain surgeon explained that the tumour had indeed been removed entirely, but that this wasn't in itself sufficient to provide a confident cure and that radiotherapy would be required as well. For his part, the radiotherapist seemed in two minds about whether or not the radiotherapy should be supplemented by chemotherapy, but eventually opted for radiation alone, explaining to Paul's mother that these tumours had a tendency to seed down the spine, and therefore treatment should include not only the brain, but the whole of the spinal cord as well. It all seemed a lot to take in, particularly since Paul's mother was a single parent with two other children (one with Down's syndrome, the other with troublesome intermittent asthma) to take care of. She was particularly concerned about the discussion of possible side-effects such as growth failure and maybe even a fall-off in Paul's school performance – but there didn't really seem to be any choice.

The treatment went well; Paul's uncle was a taxi driver and was able to fetch and carry without too much difficulty. After the surgery, Paul had been extremely floppy and cantankerous for a few weeks but seemed to improve during the radiotherapy, or at least the first part of it. Towards the end, though – it was a taxing, eight-week course of treatment – he was beginning to tire easily and spent most of his afternoons in bed.

It took the family quite a while to readjust to completion of treatment and the possibility of a more normal life again. Paul's mother found the first anniversary of his diagnosis absolutely nerve-wracking. But physically, he seemed fit enough, and the cancer never reappeared, though it was an anxious time for the whole family, particularly when follow-up visits and scans were due.

Paul's now fourteen and seems completely well; the oncologist is almost certain that he's cured now. He attends for follow-up at a special growth clinic, since he needed growth hormone injections (three times a week) from shortly after the completion of radiotherapy until a few months ago. His final height looks like being five foot seven, just two inches below the initial predicted figure. Puberty seems to have been normal, and despite being warned that he might need thyroid supplements as well, this hasn't been necessary so far. A year ago, Paul started a Saturday job in a local bike shop and seems as keen as ever on messing about with grease and crankshafts. Don't ask him to walk heel-to-toe in a straight line though – he'll still fall over.

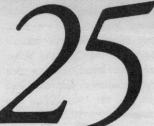

chapter
twenty-five

THE COMMONEST
QUESTIONS AND
ANSWERS

I n the bad old days, the patient used to sit there silently, hardly daring to move or breathe – all the action came from behind the consultant's desk. It wasn't the patient's business to ask too many questions! Heavens, whatever next?

But all that has changed – or, at least, in my view, it should have done. Patients have a right to know more about the treatment approaches that will affect them so profoundly: the benefits, side-effects, options, preferences – none of these are taboo subjects and for the doctor, exploration and discussion of these topics can all add up to one of the most gratifying parts of an otherwise humdrum working day.

Everyone must be aware, though – patients most particularly – that information is not only valuable but dangerous. In the search for reassurance, a patient with courage enough to ask, 'What's the chance of my being alive in a year's time?' may well receive a more gloomy response than expected – the moment's interchange altering forever his perception about his prospects, and in consequence, his priorities or choices for the future. Some relish the chance of proving the doctor wrong, others try to wish away the unwelcome news and need considerable extra support and more frequent follow-up visits.

Some of our most intelligent patients are, frankly, simply too worried about the potential side-effects treatment for their own good. This is not to deny their right to know, but the doctor has to try and ensure that their understanding is well grounded within the proper context of the potential

269

benefits and disadvantages of the treatment. I remember a highly intelligent, forty-one-year-old journalist, mother of three young children, who
read up all she could find about her tumour (including the medical
textbooks), bombarded her consultant (one of my endlessly patient
colleagues) with literally dozens of written questions, mostly of the 'What
if . . .?' variety, attended for discussion at three or four hourly sessions, then
finally refused the treatment which was clearly indicated. Less than two
months later, despite a major operation (it was the radiotherapy she
refused) the tumour had returned and – tragically too late – she now
acquiesced to his original recommendation. There comes a point where the
patient, however bright, questioning and keen to retain control, has to
invest his or her trust in the professional whose advice was sought in the first
place. It's dispiriting, of course, for an expert consultant to take a grudging
patient through treatments they would clearly prefer not to have, but far
more tragic when the opportunity for a cure is lost, simply as a result of an
unwillingness to recognise that the specialist is there to help, to be trusted
and valued. Sadly, we still see too many patients in whom an initial
opportunity for cure has passed because, for one reason or another, too little
was done too late.

The following is a collection of the dozen or so most commonly asked
questions by cancer patients, questions that have been put to me time and
time again. The answers are not intended to be – and, indeed, cannot be
– exhaustive, and they should certainly not stop you from asking your
own doctor for further information.

Is there anything I could have done to prevent the cancer?

In many cancers, we have only a very poor idea – sometimes no idea at all
– as to what was the original cause or provocation. In brain tumours,
cancers (sarcomas) of soft tissues such as muscle and cartilage, or
glandular malignancies (lymphomas), we know virtually nothing about
causation at all. No common thread has been found which defines the
type of patient most likely to develop these, though there are plenty of
fashionable, unsubstantiated theories to trap the unwary.

But, in an increasing number, we really do have some idea (see chapter
2). Lung cancer is, of course, the best example of all – the disease was
pretty unusual before smoking became popular in the early part of this
century. The link between smoking and most (but not all) forms of lung
cancer is so tight that in most studies, including those conducted at my
own hospital, over ninety per cent of lung cancer patients have smoked,
often heavily, at some time in their lives. In women who have never

smoked but are married to smokers, the risk of their developing lung cancer is over twice as great, compared with similar women who are married to non-smokers. Not surprising, perhaps – tobacco smoke contains over 4,000 different chemicals, many of which are known to be harmful. We now know that fifty per cent of all cigarette smokers will die prematurely as a result of the habit – the most important single statistic to have emerged about the evils of tobacco.

Alcohol, too, can be dangerous, and is clearly a causative factor in the head and neck cancer group (see chapter 21). In populations with a high intake of meat, the risk of cancer of the large bowel is high, and there is now a general agreement that too much meat really is bad for you – eat more fibre! As for skin cancers; the advice is to avoid too much sun (discussed more fully in chapter 18) . . . and so on.

The more we know about the causes of cancer, the more we can do to prevent their development. The current belief is that about thirty per cent of all cancer deaths are caused by smoking and that a similar figure may be related to diet, though the evidence here is much less clear. But it will certainly help to eat more fruit and vegetables, less fatty foods and meat, and avoid too much alcohol. The Health Education Council issues an excellent, free booklet entitled *Cancer – How to Reduce Your Risks*, which gives further details.

So it's a complex question, particularly where there is a genetic component – such as breast cancer, where family history is probably the most powerful in a whole variety of contributing factors. You have to choose your parents with great care! But one myth I do want to dispel is that there is a specific type of 'cancer personality'. Much has been written about this, and I think it's all nonsense. It's so easy to imagine that 'It only happens to the best people' or 'He deserved what he got', but, in my view, they are all meaningless, trivial phrases without any substance. I must have seen tens of thousands of patients with cancer, but I don't detect any particular personality or emotional features in common. Perhaps I'm just a sceptic, but I prefer to think that contentions as important as this require scientific validation. It's all too easy for devotees of this or that culture to push their pet enthusiasm.

Cancer is often regarded as a stress-related illness, since so many patients give an account of major life events which have befallen them in the months preceding the diagnosis – a broken marriage, financial disaster, death of a loved one and so on. But ask almost anyone about the last year of their life, and there'll usually be some dreadful item to relate. I've known doctors and nurses who seem to take a perverse delight in demonstrating to the patient just how their lifestyle, or recent series of personal tragedies, has burrowed into their body tissues, so to speak, and caused the cancer. Personally, I think it's wicked to make the patient feel that they're somehow to blame, though I admit it does get difficult when confronted with my twentieth new lung cancer patient in a single month, all lifelong smokers, yet touchingly keen to gain the approval of the medical team and – finally! – give up.

Should I change my diet/lifestyle to ensure the cancer doesn't return?

This is a tricky one too. As far as diet is concerned, the general points I outlined on page 271 are worth taking seriously. Try to cut down on fatty foods, meat (if you're an over-enthusiastic carnivore) and alcohol – not more than twenty-one units a week for men or fourteen for women. With some cancers (the head and neck group, stomach, liver and pancreas), it might be better to give up altogether, since alcohol may well have played a part in their causation. In any event, many patients find it easier to cut out alcohol altogether than to cut it down and keep it at a more reasonable level. Smoking is obviously best avoided – it's advice I would give to anybody anyway, though, paradoxically perhaps, I don't feel it's fair to bully certain patients about this too much – those with hopelessly incurable cancers, for example – particularly if smoking is one of their few remaining pleasures and to give up would be difficult. What's the point of stopping smoking for this unfortunate group? Sadly, it won't turn the clock back. But patients with cured head and neck cancer, for example, should be urged to stop smoking at all costs; it's a tragic fact that the commonest cause of death in patients cured of an early cancer of the larynx is a new, separate, lung cancer from continued smoking – the very same cause that was responsible for the cancer of the larynx in the first place. Every radiotherapist in the country has lost patients this way, so be sensible, eat healthily, avoid too much sun, and, if exposed to dangerous substances at work, follow the precautions about protective clothing.

As far as lifestyle is concerned, I am pretty much opposed to too much alteration here, just for the sake of it, since I don't really believe in the lifestyle theory of cancer anyway. 'Change of lifestyle' mostly means reducing your stress level, I suppose – easier said than done, it seems to me. The trouble with paying too much attention to this concept is that it's so easy for the illness to become the focus of the patient's life – change the diet, add in the vitamins, alter the lifestyle and so on – whereas I often feel a more robust attitude would be better. You've finished the treatment? You're a few years on? Good! Why not forget your previous medical history altogether, or at least push it to the margins of your life, rather than letting it continue to occupy centre stage. You've got a life to live, after all. There are more important things to do than worry about whether or not the latest food fad or trace element theory might give you an extra per cent or two in your long-term chances. Remember that the food additive industry is a multi-billion-pound affair and that cancer patients are prime and highly susceptible targets. If you eat sensibly and well – plenty of fruit, vegetables and fresh food – you won't need any additives at all. And as for reducing your stress levels to those of a hibernating sloth . . . get real! I've got more sympathy with the sentiment expressed in that wonderful line 'Don't tell me to relax, it's only my tension that's holding me together.'

Will treatment make me infertile?

Chemotherapy can certainly cause infertility, though not all the drugs do this. In young women, the risk is fairly small. On the whole, the younger the patient, the less likely she is to become infertile, presumably because the reserve store of eggs in the ovary is fixed, and the closer the patient is to her natural menopause, the more likely the chemotherapy is to completely interrupt the fertile period. Fortunately, not many women after the age of, say, forty have a continuing wish to conceive – though this, of course, can be a real issue in clinical management decisions. Even high doses of chemotherapy (of the intensity often employed with bone marrow transplantation) can be compatible with a later pregnancy – one of my patients recently produced healthy twins after just such a procedure, having suffered for ten years beforehand with a relapsing form of Hodgkin's disease.

In the case of young women treated for breast cancer, the traditional view in the past was that they should be discouraged from ever becoming pregnant again, on the grounds that the oestrogen surge which occurs during pregnancy could be extremely damaging for them and provide just the kind of environment that the cancer would exploit, developing once again in the favourable milieu. On the whole, this view is no longer taken, at least not to the same level of absolute diktat, though I do think it is right to caution women that there is a possible theoretical risk of this kind. On the whole, though, the scant evidence we have on the subject seems to be reassuring. Women who are desperate to become pregnant after treatment for breast cancer will obviously have to decide for themselves what their priorities are.

In men, chemotherapy can certainly cause infertility, the details again depending on the specifics of the drugs and the dosages used. Unlike the situation in women however, it is perfectly possible to freeze sperm and use the sample later, to inseminate the wife or partner if it becomes clear, after successful treatment for the cancer, that the patient's fertility has been damaged beyond repair. In young men treated for cancer, the issue of fertility should always be explored and sperm storage offered. There is quite a lot of evidence that many men are cured of chemo-responsive cancers without suffering permanent sterility.

Radiotherapy is a different matter. There is no risk of infertility whatsoever, provided that the gonads (the ovaries or the testicles) aren't irradiated directly, except for a very small number of patients (generally children or adolescents) in whom a course of radiotherapy for a brain tumour may damage the pituitary area. Even in these patients, however, it is generally possible to deal adequately with the problem, through simple hormone replacement, if puberty (and therefore fertility) does not occur naturally.

If radiotherapy is a necessary part of treatment, either directly to the ovaries or both testes, there is virtually no prospect of continued fertility, because of the damage directly caused to the ova (eggs) or sperm precursors. This point also applies to the large majority of patients treated by total body irradiation – usually as an adjunct to bone marrow transplantation for leukaemia or other disorders.

When cancer patients do conceive and have children (or father them), the risks of damage to the developing foetus are very small indeed, probably negligible, as a result of the cancer treatment though we do, on the whole, suggest to patients that they try and ensure an eighteen- to twenty-four-month period between the end of treatment and any attempt to conceive.

What should I do if the cancer is diagnosed when I am pregnant, or if I conceive during treatment?

Fortunately, this does not occur very often, and it's not really possible to give absolute guidance. Each individual case will depend very much on the circumstances. For example, in a women of thirty-two, with three healthy children, diagnosed with a potentially fatal, yet curable, gynae-cological cancer during the early stages of pregnancy, the strong advice of most specialists would be to allow treatment to proceed in order to cure the mother, even though this will inevitably result in termination of the pregnancy. In cancer of the cervix, for instance, where the cure rates are high if the disease is diagnosed and treated early, this must surely be the right advice. On the other hand, if the disease is diagnosed during the final stages of pregnancy, with delivery only a couple of months away, it is not so unreasonable, especially if the pregnancy is a particularly 'precious' one, to keep a very careful watch on the pregnancy, induce labour or deliver by caesarian section at the earliest safe opportunity, and then get on quickly with the normal treatment within a short time afterwards.

With chemotherapy treatments, similar difficult decisions have to be made. I remember treating a very young woman some years ago with widespread breast cancer, six months pregnant and with only a small chance of surviving herself to the expected delivery date. Chemotherapy seemed the only possible means of keeping her alive, but might it harm the baby? We did go ahead and treat her, since the obstetric advice was that the baby's organs would be fully formed already, and fortunately she gave birth to a healthy 8-pound boy just a few weeks before she herself died from this terrible disease. I wasn't sure I'd done the right thing until I was invited to the christening and learned that they'd named the child after me (the only time it's ever happened in my career) – so I think I must have done!

It's sometimes possible, though we are never terribly happy about it, to give radiotherapy during pregnancy. Another of my patients was a young research scientist who, after many unsuccessful years, had finally become pregnant. Sadly, this coincided soon afterwards with a relapse of her previously diagnosed breast cancer. She developed secondary deposits in her brain, causing partial paralysis and facial weakness. She'd initially been treated elsewhere and came to see me with her husband, both of them distraught, for a second opinion. The advice had been to terminate the pregnancy in order to allow immediate treatment. In point of fact, though, it seemed to me that one had to face the inevitability of this being a totally incurable situation – which, in her heart of hearts, she knew anyway. An immediate termination would not have turned an incurable disease into a curable one. Once she and her husband realised this, they were both adamant that the condition be treated as far as possible without a termination. Fortunately, her condition improved with steroids for the first six weeks, and radiotherapy to the brain was possible at a later stage without too much radiation dose scattering down to the pelvis (we checked this with dose monitors, of course). She, too, gave birth to a fine baby boy, and lived another four months or so. This time, they named the child after the obstetrician.

Will my hair fall out? Will it takes years to grow back?

Unfortunately, many chemotherapy drugs do cause hair loss (alopecia). Obviously the oncologist or nurse supervising your care will tell you how likely this is with the particular group of drugs that has been recommended for you. The major culprits are all discussed in chapter 5 and include doxorubicin (Adriamycin), vincristine (Cyclophosphamide), etoposide, taxol and daunorubicin – there are several more. The good news is that we can absolutely guarantee that the hair loss will be temporary (there aren't many areas in cancer medicine where we can make an absolute guarantee, so this really is quite a prize!) and that the quality of the hair, including colour, should be pretty similar to how it was previously. Quite often, the hair returns in a more 'youthful' condition – finer, silkier or more wavy. I have even had one or two partly bald men who ended up with more hair after chemotherapy than they had in the first place. It doesn't usually take all that long – there are many instances of patients regrowing hair even before completion of the chemotherapy administration. Within three months or so, hair regrowth should be very satisfactory.

Radiotherapy also affects the hair, but only when the radiation beam is directed at the skull – generally for a primary or secondary brain tumour (see chapter 13). It is surprising how many people believe that radiotherapy can cause hair loss on the scalp, even when given to a distant part of the body – chest, abdomen or pelvis. This is simply not so.

Hair recovery after radiotherapy is a more uncertain and generally slower affair than after chemotherapy. It is highly dose dependent, i.e. recovery will be much quicker after a small dose than a very large one. There are many instances where, sadly, hair regrowth is poor, even after several years, particularly at the top of the head where the radiation beam passes across the top of the skull almost tangentially, creating pockets of high dosage which are impossible to avoid. Life for the radiotherapist would be easier if the skull were shaped like a sugar-cube.

It is generally possible to mask these difficulties if there really is troublesome delay of hair regrowth, either by hair pieces or, more simply, by adjusting the hair style so that the uncovered areas are disguised. A very few patients feel so psychologically damaged, though, that they request a referral to a plastic surgeon or hair expert. There are one or two cunning techniques available, including hair transplantation or the use of an expandable device which the surgeon can fit under the hair-bearing area of the scalp, gradually increasing the volume, so that a dome of hair-bearing skin develops on the patient's scalp – some of this redundant flap then being used as a hair-bearing skin graft to cover the defective site. Although these techniques are in common use elsewhere, particularly in the USA, there (fortunately) doesn't seem to be too much demand in this country. Most patients simply learn to cope – and, in any event, life is rather easier these days, since the punks and their followers have widened the range of hair styles, including very close cropping and partial baldness, that are now considered socially acceptable: an unexpected benefit of 'yoof culture'.

Will treatment affect my sex life?

Quite likely, initially. Obviously this is one of the most complex and sensitive of issues, but there are a number of important points to make. Firstly, the news of the diagnosis itself, and the complicated psychological reactions afterwards – anger, bitterness, sadness, guilt, frustration and so on – are hardly conducive to nights of passion. This is an important point – partners have to be supportive, understanding and flexible. On the other hand, there are couples who find that the diagnosis of a life-threatening condition brings them closer in all respects (including sex), so it would be foolish to suggest hard-and-fast advice as to what might happen. As for the treatment itself, it's the sickness and debilitation following a major operation, radiotherapy or chemotherapy that is more likely to reduce your libido, rather than the specific effects of, say, the chemotherapy agents themselves. If your sex life does suffer after treatment, it's not likely to be due to any organic treatment-related cause, but it's much more frequently a totally understandable psycho-logical reaction to a highly threatening and anxiety-provoking experience. There is no reason why your sex life shouldn't return to normal afterwards, even if it has been affected during the treatment.

There are one or two caveats to this, chiefly concerning treatment by hormone therapy in men with prostate cancer. For example, radical operations can lead to impotence (though recent developments have meant that even a radical prostectomy need not always have this effect). The hormones which are often used in prostate cancer can render men impotent as well.

An equally important group for special mention includes younger women with gynaecological cancers or breast cancer, in whom treatment by surgery, radiation or chemotherapy has brought on an early meno-pause. Although this may be desirable, as, for example, in patients with breast cancer, the effects can be profound. Many patients complain bitterly about the early ageing, loss of skin, hair and general body tone and perhaps especially, loss of libido, this latter often compounded by discomfort or bleeding during intercourse as a result of the thinning of the vaginal lining. In the case of patients with gynaecological cancers suffering these troublesome side-effects, hormone replacement therapy is both safe and effective – a real life-saver in many. On the whole, there seems no reason whatever to deny women HRT, apart from the small group of pre-menopausal patients with endometrial cancer (see chapter 14) in whom oestrogen replacement is generally regarded as undesirable, since it might stimulate regrowth of the cancer. Some specialists feel the same level of concern for patients with cancer of the cervix (neck of the womb) who have an adenocarcinoma (a glandular-type cancer), which mimics, at least in its appearance under the microscope, the cancers more typically associated with the lining of the womb. Even in this group, however, it is at least possible to use progestogen drugs, such as Provera or Megace, which often give a fair degree of recovery, even though they don't contain any oestrogen; a more recently available drug, known as Tibolone (Livial), can also be helpful in this respect.

Pre-menopasual patients with breast cancer present a particular problem since, increasingly, chemotherapy is used in this group, for very good reasons but with the side-effect of producing an early menopause. Since many surgeons and other specialists believe that the induction of the early menopause is a key part of the therapeutic effect, it seems illogical to use HRT for such patients, although the traditional view has softened a little in recent years. Speaking for myself, I still feel rather concerned about its use, particularly in patients at real risk of recurrence (usually by virtue of positive axillary lymph glands). Once again, Provera, Livial or similar drugs can be extraordinarily valuable, without the potential dangers of HRT. In severe unresponding cases, however, I certainly agree that a miserable life without HRT can be so dreadful for the patient, and possibly so disruptive to her marital and sexual relationships, that HRT should be used. In my own experience, modest doses of Provera (around 20 milligrams a day) are effective in about two-thirds of all patients in reducing, or even abolishing, the menopausal effects – not bad for an agent which doesn't contain any oestrogen and seems perfectly safe both on practical and theoretical grounds.

Can we be sure the cancer is gone?
All cancers are different, and some are particularly unpredictable, capable of reappearing unexpectedly after many years when all traces had apparently been eradicated. The good news, though, is that these are less common than the large numbers in which, after five years free of recurrence of disease, one can be pretty certain that the disease will not recur. This applies to the large bulk of cancers we treat, and in a small number, one can even be pretty confident after as little as two or three

years. Testicular tumours, for example, were so vicious before today's effective treatments that they would generally reappear (if they were going to come back at all) within two years or so. With modern treatment, freedom from recurrence for a two-year period is virtually tantamount to cure. The same applies for the small cell variety of lung cancer (the type which is most closely associated with smoking), which is so malignant that recurrence after treatment is very common within two years, only a small minority of patients proving to be cured in the long run. In head and neck cancer sites, the two- to three-year rule applies once again: relapses after this time are uncommon, and follow-up visits to the clinic won't have to be so frequent, most specialists insisting on a monthly follow-up schedule during the crucial first year which represents the real danger period.

The major exception to all this is breast cancer, which is a dreadfully capricious disease, capable of lying quiescent for ten years or more, then returning quite unexpectedly. Although this might sound like an impossible, Damoclean situation, the very late relapse of this type is fortunately uncommon. Over two-thirds of breast cancer patients remain alive and well during the first five years of treatment, the majority of whom will remain disease-free at the tenth year of follow-up as well. Other conditions where relapses can occur late include melanoma (see chapter 18) and cancer of the kidney, which can also behave in a very curious way, apparently remaining under total control, without evidence of residual disease, but with late relapse as a very well-documented occasional feature.

For all these reasons, it's difficult to generalise, but, in most cases, freedom from disease at, say, the five-year mark is pretty good evidence of cure. Follow-up clinics are extremely important; they not only help the specialist to build up an ever more complete picture of you (and perhaps your family as well), but also they provide excellent opportunities for training young doctors who hope to become specialists themselves as well as the medical students who so badly need to know that cancer patients can indeed lead active, fruitful and often untroubled lives after treatment. From the patient's point of view, of course, they represent an important part of the insurance against recurrence, or at least the early recognition of recurrent disease with, hopefully, some prospect of further active treatment.

What happens if the cancer comes back?

There is an important difference between recurrence at the initial, or primary, site and recurrence at a distant site or sites (secondary deposits).

With recurrence at the primary site, it is sometimes possible to operate again, to remove the whole of the diseased area – or to offer radiotherapy, if this has not previously been done. Patients with brain tumours, cancers of the large bowel recurring at the site of the anastomosis (the area where the two cut ends of the bowel had been joined together again after the first operation to remove the tumour) and breast cancer quite often fall into this group. For many breast cancer patients these days, in whom a small local excision operation has been followed by radiotherapy, recurrence at the primary site (which occurs in about seven per cent of such patients) can be managed very successfully, though this usually means a mastectomy, or, at the very least, a wider operation than was originally performed. If, for technical reasons, surgery is no longer possible, then radiotherapy is often useful, provided it hasn't already been given to this same area.

Where the recurrence is of the rather more common secondary type, at distant sites or in local lymph node (glandular) areas, the ball game is altogether different. Local lymph node spread can sometimes be dealt with surgically, but, in general, patients with this type of recurrence are very difficult to cure. For most cancers, it isn't the primary but the secondary deposits, with their often relentless pattern of spread, that prove fatal in the end. Chemotherapy or hormone therapy are often well worthwhile, however, since they can both help to halt the progress of the secondaries. Very occasionally (but not all that often, I have to admit) it is still possible to cure patients, even at this late stage – testicular and thyroid cancers are good examples, discussed more fully in chapters 17 and 21.

Since chemotherapy can be quite a troublesome form of treatment for the patient, it can be difficult to decide whether events should be allowed to take their course, so to speak, or perhaps to take a more active line and offer chemotherapy, even in unpromising circumstances. In my view, this difficult judgement is usually best made by careful discussion with the patient, sometimes with the family as well, and deciding together what seems best. The patient certainly shouldn't be under any illusions as to what can reasonably be expected, but palliative treatment of this kind can be extremely valuable in reducing symptoms and perhaps granting the patient a few extra months or even years. Sometimes one is pleasantly surprised even in unpromising circumstances. Hormone therapies can be extremely valuable as well, though perhaps for a more limited group of diseases – cancers of the breast, prostate and uterus are the best examples. All of these may prove responsive, even if spread to distant sites has occurred, for periods of months or even years, generally with few side-effects. It is for this reason that most specialists still prefer to use hormone therapy first, before chemotherapy, in diseases such as breast cancer where either could reasonably be offered.

If the opportunity for active treatment really has passed, most patients (but not all – there aren't any hard-and-fast rules) prefer to know rather than be fobbed off. The doctor's responsibility doesn't end here, of course. A good oncologist should always be prepared to stay with the patient until the end, offering support, counselling and – perhaps most important of all – the practical advice which can be of such great help. Symptom control has advanced so much in recent years that very few patients are unresponsive to the right kind of symptom control – an enormous subject, covered more fully in chapters 5 and 7.

With me having had cancer, are my children more at risk?

On the whole, the answer to this is an unequivocal 'no'. There are very few cancers with such a strong genetic component that children will be at high risk. Perhaps the best known is the very rare childhood cancer of the eye, known as retinoblastoma, in which the genetics are very well understood; this is discussed fully in chapter 24. A much more common problem, however, is the patient with breast cancer – itself a familial disease, of course – who has a strong family history of the disease. There is no doubt that daughters of patients with breast cancer are at greater risk of developing the disease (probably about double) and that the more family members affected, the more likely the risk. No one quite knows what to do with this information, and, in the USA, the operation of bilateral prophylactic subcapsular mastectomy (i.e. removal of both breasts before there is any sign of disease, but with preservation of the skin and nipples, together with immediate reconstruction) has become a little more popular in recent years in women from high-risk families who request it. This very drastic approach has not yet taken hold in the UK or Europe, but one can understand both the ghastly logic and the terrible predicament of a young woman who knows she is at very high risk by virtue of a strong family history. It's probably sensible for such patients to be screened from an earlier age (mid-thirties, say, rather than the normal recommendation of fifty years) using mammography, which can be repeated every two years or so.

Other familial cancer syndromes are very unusual. There is a type of familial bowel disorder, characterised by multiple polyps which have a high propensity to malignant change, and, once again, screening is generally recommended for these patients, using direct vision by colonoscopy (see also chapter 2, page 7).

Families with a high incidence of ovarian cancer are also well recognised. On the whole, though, the genetic component of cancer is not sufficiently strong to represent a real threat to any offspring of cancer patients. The best advice, of course, is: don't smoke, eat sensibly, avoid too much sunlight – all the points that were covered in the answers to the first two questions.

Will my physical appearance be affected by treatment?

Internal surgery should not make any difference at all, apart from the scar, of course. Some of the most exciting advances in cancer surgery over the past decade have been based not only on technical improvements, but also on the increasing recognition that body image really is important – hence the emphasis on local excision with breast preservation, rather than mastectomy, if at all possible. Breast reconstruction is, of course, a real option for patients who are keen to have it. Surgeons vary as to the techniques they use and when they feel it should best be performed but in general, far more women are now opting to at least explore the possibility of a breast reconstruction, which can sometimes include the nipple as well. For the most part, recent scares about leakage of silicone implants seem largely without foundation, and some of the really sophisticated techniques don't rely on these implants so heavily, anyway. In malignant bone tumours, particularly those affecting the limbs in young adolescents, advances in conservative and restorative surgery have been really astonishing. Even as little as twenty years ago, amputation was almost always required, whereas we now have a whole series of bio-engineered, tailor-made internal metallic implants, some of which even have expandable shafts for growth, which allow preservation of the adult or growing limb. Speaking valves are also more widely used nowadays.

Even facial operations can often be achieved with a minimum of external scarring and deformity, since surgeons are often very expert at devising their operations to allow placement of the surgical scar in a natural fold of skin – a forehead crease or the crease which runs down the side of the nose, for example. Laryngectomy, of course, leaves a permanent stoma (hole) at the front of the neck, but this is usually disguised by a small pad which is porous enough to allow for breathing (that's the point of the stoma, of course), and a collar and tie will often disguise most of this, anyway. Speaking valves are also more widely used nowadays.

I have already discussed the issue of hair loss from radiotherapy and chemotherapy. In other respects, neither of these treatments should cause permanent scarring or change of body image, though high doses of radiotherapy can sometimes lead to subtle skin changes which may be permanently visible – small leashes of tiny veins, or areas of additional or deficient pigmentation. On the whole, these shouldn't be too marked with normal radiation techniques – unless, of course, the site has to be re-irradiated because of local recurrence, though radiotherapists are always very cautious about this. Radiotherapy can also lead to permanent loss of body hair in the site irradiated (armpit, pubic area, chest and so on), though very few patients are at all bothered about this – it's often seen as rather a boon.

Everyone's been so supportive – why do I feel so awful?

This is a very common question, probably more often unvoiced than spoken aloud. It's terribly common for patients to feel they've 'let the side down' by not picking themselves up, dusting themselves down and simply getting on with it. The truth, of course, is that support from friends, families and the medical, nursing and other staff is all important, but – and it's a big but – you the patient don't have to feel obliged in some way, as if you have your own side of a contractual bargain to keep. If everyone's being warm and wonderful, well, great; but it may well not lessen, or at least not abolish, the hurt, the injury and the fear which inevitably strike even the most detached and cool-headed of patients. You are not some kind of machine, inevitably reaching the right kind of emotional response to the extra degree of support that may well come your way. You may well feel, despite a dispassionate appreciation, an additional sense of frustration that you somehow owe it to those around you to behave better. Don't, though – rise above it, and recognise the love and the concern for what they are, without feeling that they, the givers, have any real right to press a few of your emotional buttons and expect you blithely to snap out of it in some straightforward, mechanistic way. Perhaps I'm even suggesting it's a time to be selfish, though you may not normally be one to place yourself centre stage. You've enough on your plate already without putting on a brave face if you aren't ready to do so. It'll probably happen anyway, when you least expect it, and at a later point in your life – the sudden realisation that, quite of the blue, you are beginning to feel your old self again. It's like responding to another's love, however fervently offered – you just can't force it.

Most people are able to pick up the pieces in the end, and those with support from friends, family, lovers are the lucky ones, I suppose, even though these cohorts of well-wishers can sometimes make you feel additionally burdened. Certainly the volumes of advice (often about treatment, diet, lifestyle and so on) offered by the supporting cast can be extremely difficult for patients to deal with, particularly where it conflicts with what they have been told by the professionals looking after them. It can be extremely discomforting for patients, who may initially feel content with the professional advice but become increasingly uncertain that the doctor is acting in their best interests, if additional dietary and other advice, well meant of course by the friends and relations, wasn't recommended by the specialist in the first place. Quite often the best I feel I can do for patients bombarded with advice, the telephone ringing all day and half the night, is to tell them to be tough and explain to all these well-meaning people that you've been told to rest more – blame it on the doctor, for heaven's sake – and get off the phone if you don't feel up to talking! You don't owe it to anyone to behave like a professional patient, constantly grateful for all they're doing, etc. You can always make it up to them later if you really feel that badly about it.

For many patients, this dreadful episode of their lives can be transmuted later into remarkable new insights, new visions of what really is important. It may sound platitudinous to talk in this context about the beauty of so much in the world around us, the poignancy of friendships, the enjoyment of some of the more simple pleasures of life, but I've heard these statements too often to simply dismiss them in the cruel, over-sophisticated manner which doctors can sometimes unwittingly adopt. For many patients recovering slowly from cancer's appalling assault on their lives, these issues are real, vibrant and comforting.

The oncologist tells me it's a 'low-grade' tumour, so I shouldn't worry too much. What on earth's he talking about?

This is quite a common question too. Try as we might, doctors sometimes find it difficult to avoid using jargon of this type – I suppose all professional groups are much the same. Tumour grading is a term used to describe the inherent growth characteristics of cancers; this is done by careful microscopic examination in the pathology lab of the tissue which was removed or sampled by biopsy. Under the microscope, low-grade tumours sometimes appear not all that different from the normal tissues they arise from, whereas the higher-grade cancers look much more disordered, even bizarre. Most tumours show characteristics of either low, intermediate or high grade, a single variety rather than a jumble; though, of course, there can be exceptions to this general rule.

The importance of grading is that the clinician in charge of a patient can use the information to help assess the severity of each case and, to some extent, predict both its likely speed of evolution and general clinical behaviour. Low-grade tumours are often much more indolent than the higher grades: brain tumours and non-Hodgkin lymphomas are good examples (see chapters 13 and 19). For these tumours, pathological grade largely determines the choice of treatment. Low-grade lymphoma, for instance, may not require treatment at all (at least in the initial stages, which may last for many years, even after a firm diagnosis has been made), whereas high-grade lymphoma in a young, fit person inevitably requires combination chemotherapy and sometimes even a bone marrow transplant with intensive drug treatment and total body irradiation.

How will I feel mentally and emotionally during the treatment?

Every patient reacts differently. For some, it's business as usual, all the way through. Others, on the other hand, find the whole business of diagnosis and treatment so distressing that the utmost reassurance and support seem to make little impact. For the most part, patients seem to cope remarkably well – possibly, I've always thought, because the initial diagnosis is so upsetting that the knowledge that treatment is indeed available, coupled with the concern and professional expertise of the staff, is itself extremely therapeutic. Some years ago, a research team looking at breast cancer patients found that they could roughly divide them into four groups: those with 'fighting spirit', who mentally and physically rose to the challenge, so to speak; then at the other end of the emotional spectrum were those who were 'stoic acceptors' of the illness; in between was the 'helpless, hopeless' group, and finally the 'denyers', who put the whole affair to one side, as it were, and simply dismissed it in order to get on with their lives.

Although the work has remained controversial, it's always struck a chord for me, since many oncologists would, I think, recognise these responses. The really contentious part of the research was the suggestion that the personality characteristics might have a bearing on outcome, since two of these groups of patients seemed to do far better than the others. Interestingly, it was the first and last groups (the denyers and those with fighting spirit) who did well, the others much less so. Not perhaps what one might have expected, though quite what one makes of this research is not at all clear – it's no easy matter to alter one's emotional responses, let alone one's personality!

Most patients feel well supported during the treatment itself, particularly since so many of the unpleasant, treatment-related symptoms can now be dealt with quite effectively by anti-nauseants, attention to skin care and so on. It is often much more difficult in the first weeks following completion of treatment, as if the sudden transition from intensive activity and clinic visits to a far more detached follow-up protocol is akin to being cast adrift on a choppy sea. Depression and anxiety are probably far more common during this period than during the treatment itself, often totally unrecognised both by the medical staff and the patient's family. What often makes it worse is that the patient often feels so guilty at this point – just at the time when champagne corks should be popping, he may possibly feel at his lowest ebb. Families and loved ones need to be particularly aware of this to avoid falling into the 'After all they've done for you . . . It's time to snap out of it' scenario. The truth, of course, is that the process of rehabilitation and re-entry into a normal lifestyle is only just beginning.

Will I be able to continue working during treatment?

Tricky one, this. On the whole, yes. Strange to say, most people actually seem to enjoy their work – some even find it quite therapeutic to continue or resume normal activities, so to speak, rather than sit around at home, frustrated, bored and introspective. For many of us, work provides not only a degree of satisfaction, but also self-esteem – and the support of colleagues who provide, at the very least, a reminder of normality and may sometimes have been through the same thing themselves. The traditional view of enforced rest from work as an essential part of recovery has largely gone by the board, though obviously circumstances will vary. Some types of work are physically too strenuous for a weakened patient to cope with, and some, such as teaching, may be too exposed or demanding; the ideal, perhaps, is a flexible arrangement whereby the patient can go in part time, or perhaps take a few weeks or months off entirely, before resuming part time in the first instance. In really high-pressure jobs, it may be best to withdraw entirely – one of my medical colleagues, a consultant surgeon with cancer, told me that he found it extremely odd not to get up at 6.30 a.m. every day and be in the operating theatre by 7.45, and had real difficulty during the first fortnight dealing with his feelings of guilt and lowered self-esteem. After that, however, he saw it quite differently as the opportunity of a lifetime! It certainly makes many re-think their work patterns, and although the majority wish to resume as normal, some patients see their professional or working lives in a totally new perspective.

Most forms of cancer treatment are tiring – particularly, perhaps, an extended course of radiotherapy. You shouldn't underestimate this – it can be a potent cause of irritability and disenchantment if you attempt to return at full tilt too soon. Perhaps the hardest part is to recognise just how much you're capable of, pace yourself a bit, but don't expect yourself to perform at full capacity straight away. The tendency is to prove to the world that you're absolutely back to normal in record time – try to resist!

What are my chances of survival and making a full recovery?

Every patient has the right to ask this, though not all wish to. Not everybody wants to put the doctor on the spot, so to speak, or to risk hearing an unwelcome reply. As I mentioned earlier in the book, a difficult situation can arise when a patient chooses not to ask this highly charged question him or herself but their spouse or partner does it for them, leaving the oncologist uncertain as to whether the patient would wish to voice the question at all. Personally, I think there is something rather improper about responding, unless it is clear that the patient (not just the spouse or companion) really does want to have the information.

I have tried in the disease-specific chapters to give a reasonable account of the prospects for recovery for most of the main types of cancer, and there certainly isn't space here to recapitulate too fully. However, for cancers that have remained localised at their point of origin, and are generally surgically removable or successfully treatable by radiotherapy, the chances of recovery are often high – over ninety per cent, for example, in the case of a small cancer of the larynx treated by radiotherapy, with full preservation of the normal voice and powers of speech. In other cancers, with a higher tendency for spread, the outlook is obviously less certain but even in these, modern research has increasingly provided methods for recognising the potential for tumour dissemination and, to some extent, pre-empting it – breast cancer is probably the best example, in which both chemotherapy and hormone treatments can be used prophylactically to lower the risk of this occurring. We now recognise that this can also be achieved, to some extent, with another large group of tumours – the colorectal (large bowel) cancers. The likelihood of recovery is determined not only by the details of anatomic sites of disease (the tumour stage), but also, as mentioned above, the pathological character-istics (tumour grade), as well as other factors, such as the chromosomal content of the malignant cells, the molecular cell markers, which can be determined by special staining methods in the laboratory, and the presence of tumour extension to local lymph node groups. All these points are both important and predictive of the outcome, yet we still fall far short of the ideal – an accurate determination of the prognosis for each patient, which at the very least would allow us to tailor our intensity of treatment with much greater confidence. For some tumours, particularly those which are chemo-sensitive, the completeness of the chemotherapy response is so important as a predictive factor for outcome that it may outweigh all other considerations – an observation which has led some oncologists to the conclusion that winding up the dose of chemotherapy might represent the most promising form of novel cancer therapy for partly responsive tumours. Quite a number of trial groups are investigating this at present.

SUMMARY

Inevitably, many other questions arise, particularly in relation to specific areas which I have tried to anticipate and deal with in more detail in chapters 11 to 24.

All specialists are busy, sometimes rushed off their feet, but most are only too willing to try and answer questions. Do be ready with them, though – the amount of time available will inevitably be limited, and you will naturally want to use it in the best possible way. There is no point in pretending, though, that one can predict the future with complete accuracy, so don't be surprised if some of the replies are somewhat guarded. Living with uncertainty may be the most difficult part of the whole illness, but facing up to both the facts and the limitations of what we know is undoubtedly the best means of regaining some sort of control over your affairs. Good luck!

USEFUL ADDRESSES

ENGLAND

BACUP
121/123 Charterhouse Street
London
EC1M 6AA
Tel:
(Cancer Information Service)
0171 608 1661
(Freeline, from outside London)
0800 181199
(Counselling Service)
0171 608 1038

BCMA (Breast Care and Mastect-
omy Association of Great Britain)
15/19 Britten Street
London
SW3 3TZ
Tel:
Helpline: 0171 867 1103
Administration: 0171 867 8275

British Association for Counselling
1 Regent Place
Rugby
CV21 2PJ

British Colostomy Association
15 Station Road
Reading
Berkshire
RG1 1LG
Tel: 01734 391537

CARE (Cancer Aftercare and
Rehabilitation Society)
21 Zetland Road
Redland
Bristol
BS6 7AH
Tel: 01272 427419

CancerLink
17 Britannia Street
London
WC1X 9JN
Tel: 0171 833 2451

Cancer Relief Macmillan Fund
Anchor House
15/19 Britten Street
London
SW3 3TZ
Tel: 0171 351 7811

Carers' National Association
29 Chilworth Mews
London
W2 3RG
Tel: 0171 724 7776

The Cinnamon Trust (for pet care
whilst patients are in hospital)
Poldarves Farm
Trescowe Common
Penzance
Cornwall
TR20 9RX
Tel: 01736 850291

CRUSE – Bereavement Care
Cruse House
126 Sheen Road
Richmond
Surrey
TW9 1UR
Tel: 0181 940 4818

Hodgkin's Disease Association
PO Box 275
Haddenham
Aylesbury
Bucks
HP17 8JJ
Tel: 01844 291500
(9am–10pm, 7 days)

Hospice Information Service
St. Christopher's Hospice
51–59 Lawrie Park Road
Sydenham
London
SE26 6DZ
Tel: 0181 778 9252

Hysterectomy Support Network
3 Lynne Close
Green Street Green
Orpington
Kent
BR6 6BS
Tel: 0181 856 3881
(answerphone)

The Institute for Complementary
Medicine
PO Box 194
London
SE16 1QZ
Tel: 0171 237 5165

The Institute of Family Therapy
43 New Cavendish Street
London
W1M 7RG
Tel: 0171 935 1651

The Leukaemia Care Society
14 Kingfisher Court
Venny Bridge
Pinhoe
Exeter
Devon
EX4 8JN
Tel: 01392 64848

Leukaemia Research Fund
(Research Body)
43 Great Ormond Street
London
WC1N 3JJ
Tel: 0171 405 0101

Lymphoma Research Trust
(Research Body)
(Funding Charity of the BNLI)
c/o BNLI
The Middlesex Hospital
Mortimer Street
London
W1N 8AA

The Malcolm Sargent Cancer
Fund For Children
14 Abingdon Road
London
W8 6AF
Tel: 0171 937 4548

Marie Curie Cancer Care
28 Belgrave Square
London
SW1X 8QG
Tel: 0171 235 3325

The National Association of
Laryngectomee Clubs
Ground Floor
6 Rickett Street
Fulham
London
SW6 1RU
Tel: 0171 381 9993

NHS (National Health Service)
Health Benefits Division
Sandyford House
Newcastle upon Tyne
NE2 1DB

The Neuroblastoma Society
Neville and Jane Oldridge
Woodlands
Ordsall Park Road
Retford
Notts.
DN22 7PJ
Tel: 01777 709238

Oesophageal Patients' Association
16 Whitefields Crescent
Solihull
West Midlands
B91 3NU
Tel: 0121 704 9860

Retinoblastoma Society
Margaret Atkin
c/o Childrens Department
Moorfields Eye Hospital
City Road
London
EC1V 2PD
Tel: 0171 253 3411 ex.2345

The Sue Ryder Foundation
Cavendish
Sudbury
Suffolk
CO10 8AY
Tel: 01787 280252

Urostomy Association
(Central Office)
"Buckland"
Beaumont Park
Danbury
Essex
CM3 4DE
Tel: 01245 224294

IRELAND

Irish Cancer Society
Information Officer
5 Northumberland Road
Dublin 4
Tel: Dublin (011) 681855
Helpline: Dublin (011) 681233

The Ulster Cancer Foundation
40–42 Eglantine Avenue
Belfast
BT9 6DX
Tel: 01232 663281/2/3
Helpline: 01232 663439
(9.30–12.30 weekdays)

SCOTLAND

Breast Care and Mastectomy
Association
Suite 2/8 65 Bath Street
Glasgow
G2 2BX
Tel: 0141 353 1050

Cancer Relief Macmillan Fund
9 Castle Terrace
Edinburgh
EH1 2DP
Tel: 0131 229 3276

CancerLink
(address as above)
Tel: 0131 228 5557

Tak Tent
Cancer Support Organisation
G Block
Western Infirmary
Glasgow
G11 6NT
Tel: 0141 334 6699/357 4519

WALES

Tenovus Cancer Information
Centre
142 Whitchurch Road
Cardiff
CF4 3NA
Tel: 01222 619846
Helpline: 01222 691998
(9am–5pm Mon Fri;
answerphone at other times)

INDEX